STRETCHING
Basics

D0710112

STRETCHING
Basics

Roberto Maccadanza

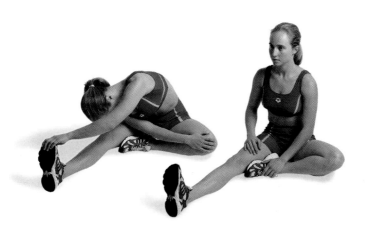

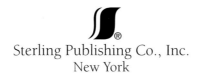

Sterling Publishing Co., Inc.
New York

Appreciation and thanks go to the following people for their collaboration with the photographs:
Valentina Volpe, Linda Perina, Anna Dall'Ora, Francesca Carpene, and Francesca Maccadanza.

Special thanks to Benessereglobale Centro Wellness

Dedicated to my parents Edda and Cesarino.

Library of Congress-in-Publication Data Available

10 9 8 7 6 5 4 3 2 1

Published in 2004 by Sterling Publishing Co., Inc.
387 Park Avenue South, New York, NY 10016
Originally published in Italy in 2001 under the title *Stretching e Stretching* by
Giunti Gruppo Editoriale S.p.A.
via Bolognese 165-50139, Firenze, Italy
Copyright © 2001 by Giunti Guppo Editoriale S.p.A.
English translation copyright © 2004 by Sterling Publishing Co., Inc.
Distributed in Canada by Sterling Publishing
$^{C}/_{o}$ Canadian Manda Group, One Atlantic Avenue, Suite 105,
Toronto, Ontario, Canada M6K 3E7
Distributed in Great Britain by Chrysalis Books PLC
The Chrysalis Building, Bramley Road, London W10 6SP, England
Distributed in Australia by Capricorn Link (Australia) Pty Ltd.
P.O. Box 704, Windsor, NSW 2756, Australia

Printed in China
All Rights Reserved

Sterling ISBN 1-4027-1139-5

Contents

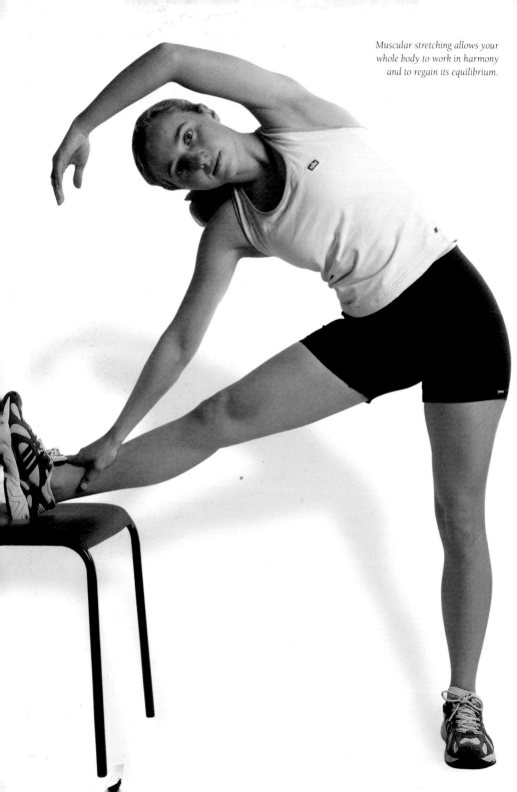

Muscular stretching allows your whole body to work in harmony and to regain its equilibrium.

What Is Stretching?

There are many exercises and workout programs to choose from to get your body into shape. However, the one activity that lies at the root of them all, and which provides the foundation for correct development, is that of *muscular extension*—commonly known as *stretching*.

Team sports, like soccer, basketball, and baseball, as well as those geared to individuals, like track, swimming, and gymnastics, all make stretching part of their conditioning regimens. Stretching is a fundamental practice that allows for the continual development of whatever athletic goal one chooses to pursue. Moreover, it is beneficial for everyone—even those who have not undertaken extensive physical training. Some of its benefits are as follows:

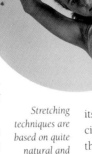

Stretching techniques are based on quite natural and everyday movements.

—**Stress relief** from problems related to physical activity and muscular development, as well as muscular and tendonal traumas such as tears and strains.

—**Improved time management**, which in turn leads to physical benefits gained by sports activity and training.

—**An awareness of your own true potential**: facing one's personal limits and, in turn, finding the means to overcome these limits.

—**The prevention of degenerative conditions** like rheumatism and osteoporosis that affect more and more people.

Later in the text, we shall explore many other such benefits—allowing you to get to know and appreciate the kind of activity that gives you the chance to achieve lasting (and often) unexpected results.

STRETCHING FOR RELAXATION

For those who know little about stretching, it is a good idea to refer to yoga. This discipline has very ancient origins; in fact, it could be defined as the "mother of stretching," insofar as it seeks control over one's own sensations, pays close attention to the body's reactions, and cultivates heightened awareness of the body and its every movement while performing an exercise. These are the same fundamental concepts that are applied to this new discipline, which we are about to discover together, and of which we hope you will gain a deeper understanding.

Stretching is a practice intimately related to the essence of being human and to our natural inclination to move—which the great majority of us allow to lie dormant. The importance of our physicality and the need to move in our daily lives has been sidetracked by our reliance on technology and our mental capacities, which limits who we are. We dull and even lose an important instinctive faculty, which is that of stretching out our bodies, just as domestic animals do; at times, we envy their ability to achieve a state of rest and repose so easily, with the simple gestures that constitute stretching. To stretch out fully, to lengthen and relax oneself: these are all related, and combine to create a fundamental basis upon which the stretching regimen rests.

Each of us can recall the pleasure of stretching out freely. We associate this with relaxation and the absence of tension, which, for example, a vacation or holiday may provide,

ignore your own well-being.

We can now acquire the much sought-after guidelines for activities directly related to stretching and learn how to apply them under various conditions, ranging from the simpler situations of everyday life to ones that are for the most part linked to physical activity, such as sport. All this will enter into the everyday movements of our lives and in turn will be added to our wealth of personal knowledge and experience.

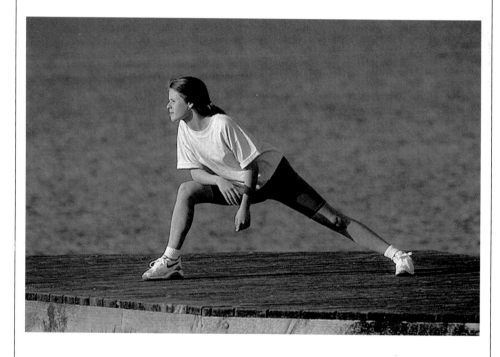

when one can be seen comfortably relaxing on the shores of the sea or awakening on a holiday morning without the urgency of going to work.

On the other hand, it is distressing to call up a memory linked with the impossibility of being able to relax freely because of a particular impediment—when a teacher didn't accept you, or after three consecutive hours of being stuck at the bank, or even worse, because good manners demand that you

RETURNING TO THE ORIGINS

Recovering the origins of stretching has not been a one-man task, even if we can attribute its popularity and worldwide circulation to the work of one Bob Anderson in 1980. He was the first to compile a text of much of the pertinent information that still constitutes such a large part of modern sports; his findings have been applied to various athletic fields and are respected in gyms in all over the world.

The birth of the practice known as *muscular elongation* (before being labeled by the vast majority simply as "stretching") is somewhat difficult to account for historically. Long ago, man and beast stretched in a very natural way, without following precise procedures.

As already mentioned, yoga can be considered the precursor of what we today call modern stretching. The first yoga postures were found stamped on the surface of rock

by many westerners in their gyms. This graceful discipline is noteworthy for the harmony and elegance it elicits in its adherents.

ESSENTIAL CONCEPTS LINKED TO MOTOR ACTIVITY

Recent research and statistics have helped us learn more about the relationship between humans and motor activity (i.e., exercising). These studies have divided their subjects into

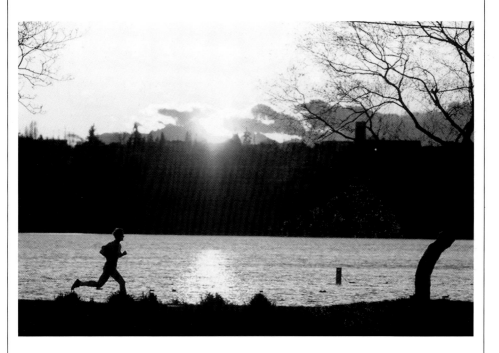

seals in the Indus Valley region and date back to around 3000 B.C. Other activities of oriental origin have emphasized psychological, spiritual, and physical equilibrium in order to improve the body's flexibility and agility with respect to strength, resistance, and increase of muscle mass. Among many others we may single out Tai Chi Chuan, which is still practiced today by the Chinese in the city squares of their towns as well as

the following three clearly defined categories:

—People who would like to exercise but lack the will and leisure time, and who, owing to fatigue, have decided to exercise in a way that makes them sweat: this they usually do in midsummer when it is 100 degrees in the shade;

—Those who dedicate themselves to sport as the utmost expression of their way of life, their

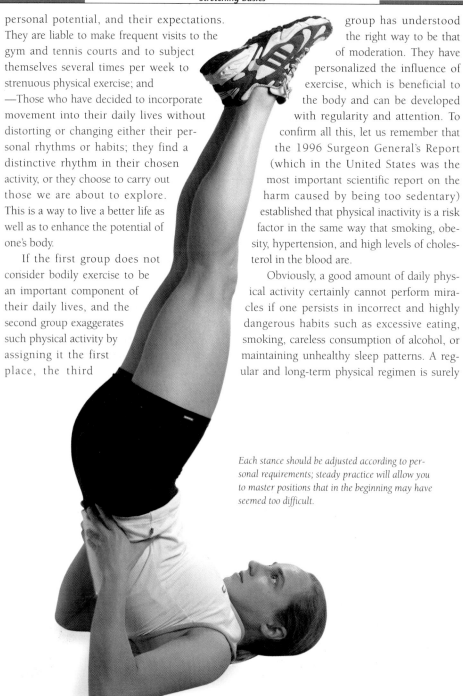

personal potential, and their expectations. They are liable to make frequent visits to the gym and tennis courts and to subject themselves several times per week to strenuous physical exercise; and

—Those who have decided to incorporate movement into their daily lives without distorting or changing either their personal rhythms or habits; they find a distinctive rhythm in their chosen activity, or they choose to carry out those we are about to explore. This is a way to live a better life as well as to enhance the potential of one's body.

If the first group does not consider bodily exercise to be an important component of their daily lives, and the second group exaggerates such physical activity by assigning it the first place, the third

group has understood the right way to be that of moderation. They have personalized the influence of exercise, which is beneficial to the body and can be developed with regularity and attention. To confirm all this, let us remember that the 1996 Surgeon General's Report (which in the United States was the most important scientific report on the harm caused by being too sedentary) established that physical inactivity is a risk factor in the same way that smoking, obesity, hypertension, and high levels of cholesterol in the blood are.

Obviously, a good amount of daily physical activity certainly cannot perform miracles if one persists in incorrect and highly dangerous habits such as excessive eating, smoking, careless consumption of alcohol, or maintaining unhealthy sleep patterns. A regular and long-term physical regimen is surely

Each stance should be adjusted according to personal requirements; steady practice will allow you to master positions that in the beginning may have seemed too difficult.

Stretching need not be a competition against oneself or others, as much as a search for and delight in the profound and pleasing sensations experienced while executing the exercises.

a worthwhile tool to begin modifying faulty rhythms of life. However, as healthy habits improve our daily life efficiency, over time it is hoped that our predisposition and capacity to practice physical activities that are good for us will increase significantly.

EFFECTS OF PHYSICAL EXERCISE

To better understand the importance of physical exercise—and in particular that of stretching—it is necessary to explain its effects on the human body. Above all, it is useful to point out that the consequences of physical activity, and of stretching in particular, are synergistic; that is, they take in both the physical sphere as well as the psychological one.

Starting with the principal systems of the organism (i.e., the respiratory and circulatory), we will briefly analyze what other effects manifest themselves in the person who sets himself or herself the task of bodywork using the techniques of stretching.

The Respiratory System

Physical exercise enhances, in an easily observable way, the organs comprising the cardiovascular system, which are responsible for supplying the body with oxygen. Such stimulation makes itself evident in an increase of respiratory movement (inhalation and exhalation), and improves the function of organs directly related to these processes (e.g., lungs, bronchioles, veins). The various stretching procedures (explained later) will, by stimulating the respiratory organs, induce them to behave in a beneficial manner.

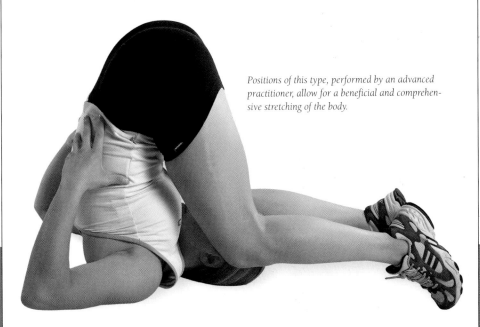

Positions of this type, performed by an advanced practitioner, allow for a beneficial and comprehensive stretching of the body.

The Circulatory System

The heart is the integral center of a closed system consisting of veins, arteries, and capillaries. It has the task of pumping oxygenated blood to the various parts of the body requiring energy, especially during the rigors of a workout.

The cardiac (heart) muscle can react to the body's increased need for energy in two different ways: one is inefficient, characterized by rapid heartbeat (a state in which the heart does not have time to refuel completely, and so starts pumping out small but regular quantities of blood). The other is more efficient—being directed by the increase in cardiac blood flow and not by the frequency of heartbeats, the result being a minimum of work and a maximum pumping of blood at each contraction.

The first state is typical of people who are not in shape, whereas the second is characteristic of those who exercise regularly. This healthful state brings in its wake a beneficial increase in cardiac activity and the prevention of pathologies brought on by leading a sedentary life.

As vein walls contract, stretching improves the cardiovascular efficiency of the muscles that move the blood toward the heart; these muscles in turn become more elastic and permit better blood flow. This process also assists in the circulation of the lymph—a substance produced by certain glands in which are immersed white blood cells, which protect the body from invasion by viruses and bacteria.

The Skeletal System

Movement stimulates bone growth generally, and, with proper nutrition, reinforces and increases bones' resistance to trauma. Stretching stimulates bone structures via the revolving action of the tendons during pulling exercises, and decreases tension accumulated by the bones through specific activities like running, sit-ups, or pull-ups.

The Muscular System

Movement induces notable changes within the muscles; it modifies the body both esthetically and functionally, making it work more economically and giving it elasticity and increased resistance to illness. Progressive exercise leads to an increase in the number of muscle fibers and capillaries, which helps the body store nutrients and heightens stamina.

Stretching brings to the muscles maximal supporting strength by efficiently eliminating waste products, in the form of lactic acid, that such muscular activity brings. It also eliminates muscle tension, which may eventually lead to the ailment known as arthritis. Middle age often brings with it muscle stiffening, and stretching can provide a valid defense against the loss of mobility.

Joints

Physical exercise acts upon the joints and their components (ligaments and the materials that coat the surface of joints and the joints themselves), making them more efficient. Movement stimulates the production of synovial fluid (the binding substance present within the joints), which allows for efficient functioning, rendering the ligaments elastic and resistant.

The act of stretching improves the joints, upgrading their level of mobility and degree of function, thereby creating a better dynamic within the entire body.

The Digestive System

Physical activity improves the digestive and secretory processes. During such activity, the intestine and liver carry out a variety of extremely important metabolic processes, such as the transformation of sugars into glycogen, the conversion of lactic acid (a by-product of the muscles after a workout) into glycogen, and the regulation of blood flow to the heart—all of which allow for a good workout.

Stretching while breathing from the

In time, you will feel more relaxed, which will improve your general disposition.

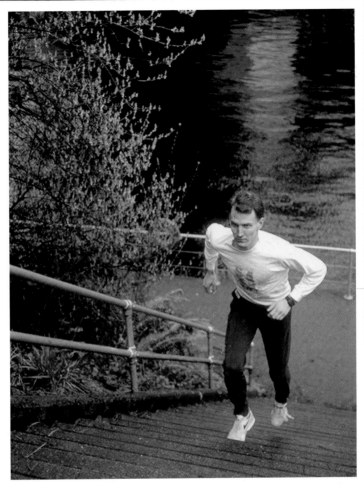

diaphragm noticeably improves digestion by increasing intestinal function. The elasticity that stretching confers on the abdominal muscles provides relief to those who suffer from constipation.

The Nervous System

Physical exercise enhances one's quality of movement, making it more economical, efficient, and coordinated. One acquires automatic responses that gain in importance on the athletic level and that notably improve the reaction times of the senses (hearing, sight, touch, and balance).

Since we must, when stretching, pay attention to what is happening to us at the physical level, we start to develop an intuitive sense of how to move, setting up exercise patterns that are both economical and coordinated. In time, a greater feeling of relaxation will permeate the entire body—a positive process that tends to improve one's general disposition.

Psychological Equilibrium

There exists a strong correlation between motor activity and mental activity. Indeed, the very close relationship between intellectual accomplishment and movement is manifested in large part during infancy, when we see their effect on the imagination, the receptive faculties, and the memory. Movement increases intellectual productivity, mental flexibility, and response to stimuli.

Motor activity can be reduced to the transfer of brain stimuli—in which the intelligence plays an active part—to accomplish particular movements. Dr. Howard Gardner, a professor of psychology at Harvard University, defines intelligence as "kinesthetic," that is, characterized by a coordination of movements that involve diverse intellectual functions and that are, at bottom, what defines us as human beings.

The emotional states of joy, happiness, sadness, and stress/strain are stimulated and controlled through movement, which makes it possible to establish one's personal equilibrium either in sports or in daily life; a run or a swim serve to "unwind" or "let off steam" after a stressful day at work. Knowing how to gauge one's own capacity, and how to manage and direct it, permits those with low self-esteem who experience unnecessary strain and tension (for whatever reason) to feel at last alive and hopeful, and to regain their own meaningful role in society.

REGULATING PHYSICAL ACTIVITY

Putting together an ongoing program of physical exercise is the first step you must take regarding your desire to obtain significant changes in your daily life. This recommendation applies to everyone, regardless of sex or age. With the swift advances of technology and the lack of green open spaces in the cities, children are increasingly confined to their apartments, where the opportunity to move is very limited. On the same note, the elderly rarely have the possibility of maintaining their state of good health through the years.

The fundamentals upon which one should base a program of physical activity are the following:

—Aerobic and cardiovascular workouts;

—A variety of strengthening exercises;

—Exercises geared to the joints that increase flexibility and mobility.

These three aspects of training should be a part of every physical training session, to a varying extent, and appropriate exercises should be tailored to the ability and limits of each individual.

▶ **Aerobic and cardiovascular** capacity means being able to handle light to moderate exertion for prolonged periods of time. Such activity can be as simple as walking up a flight of stairs, riding a bicycle, or running to catch a bus; or it may be as involved as cross-country skiing.

▶ **Strength** is the capacity of the muscles to exert force. Such power is dependent on specific groupings of the muscles. Strengthening them consists of inverting the natural process, which lessens muscle mass and increases the quantity of body fat. This starts to to occur in most persons between the ages of 25 and 30.

▶ **Joint isolation exercises** play an important part in numerous activities in daily life, as well as in the technical and sport fields. Isolation can be defined as the "ability of individual joints to function at their optimal potential." Such processes become more complex as flexibility levels increase.

▶ **Flexibility** has a similar complexity that depends on the efficiency of joint movement; also, the level of coordination and the elasticity of muscles, tendons, and ligaments must be considered. The *elastic capacity* of the muscles and their correct development through athletic work consists of helping the joints to learn a wide range of movements: the ability to twist, flex, and extend, both naturally and skillfully.

The sedentariness of our times has brought with it (in addition to many other negative effects) the progressive loss of elasticity, and consequently, a heightened risk of muscle tearing and excessive tension. Under this duress, the body naturally follows a principle of adaptation; if one sits for ten hours a day and does not stimulate the system with movements that allow for elasticity, the body will degenerate progressively until such physical lassitude becomes the norm.

Flexibility in fact depends on the elasticity of the connective and muscle tissue, and can be obtained, improved, and maintained by participation in a range of activities. Among these, stretching has an important place.

15

Muscles and Movement

The muscles, viewed as a group, comprise the *muscular system*, and can rightly be compared to a specialized machine capable of transforming chemical energy (obtained indirectly through the breaking down of sugars and fats) into mechanical energy.

Muscle can be classified in three ways: as smooth muscle, skeletal (striated) muscle, and cardiac muscle.

▶ Smooth muscles are also given the name *involuntary* because they almost always function in an independent fashion. These muscles line the walls of the digestive system, and are located in the respiratory and urogenital organs.

▶ Cardiac muscle occupies a unique place, given that it functions in a specialized way; while structurally it is striated, it is nevertheless endowed with its own features—self-contracting and rhythmic, it can maintain itself even under conditions where, for instance, the stimuli become somehow harmful or threatening.

▶ The skeletal or striated muscles comprise a large portion of the musculature. They are also termed *voluntary* because they are consciously controlled and react rapidly to stimuli that arise from the central nervous system (CNS).

Skeletal muscles are bound to the body through a very strong network of fibers or "cords" known as tendons. The muscles are formed by the union of many bundles of long fibers that are yoked to the bone across the tendons.

Each muscle fiber is immersed in a liquid that contains mitochondria within it (mitochondria are intracellular organelles that contain enzymes for cell metabolism), along with myoglobin, a substance that captures oxygen from the blood and directs it to the muscle fibers. Lastly come the myofibrils, which are the most

1-2 *The smooth muscle is composed of long cells arranged in sheaves, each with its own nucleus (A). Within the intestine, a circular internal bundle produces (B) ring-like constructions, while an external longitudinal sheaf (C) generates wave-like (peristaltic) motions. Controlled by the autonomic nervous system, the contraction of the smooth muscle is involuntary.*
3-4 *Cardiac muscle is formed from branch-like cells, which contain several nuclei (D). It is organized in thick bands and arranged into spirals (E) within the ventricles of the heart, where rapid and rhythmic contractions are carried out. These rhythms are controlled by an internal regulating mechanism.*
5-6 *The skeletal muscle involves a degree of conscious control, which is why it is also termed voluntary. Composed of long cells that measure up to 14 inches (35 cm), each cell contains many nuclei and sheaves of myofibrils. It is capable of rapid contractions but tires easily.*

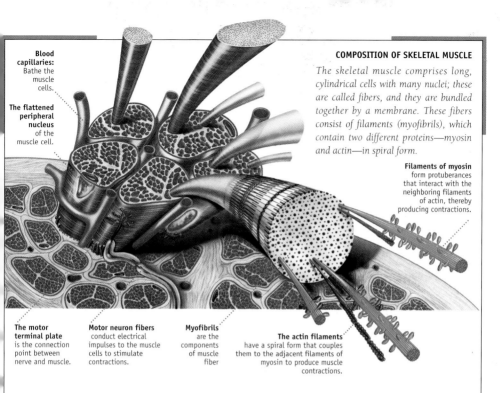

Blood capillaries: Bathe the muscle cells.

The flattened peripheral nucleus of the muscle cell.

COMPOSITION OF SKELETAL MUSCLE

The skeletal muscle comprises long, cylindrical cells with many nuclei; these are called fibers, and they are bundled together by a membrane. These fibers consist of filaments (myofibrils), which contain two different proteins—myosin and actin—in spiral form.

Filaments of myosin form protuberances that interact with the neighboring filaments of actin, thereby producing contractions.

The motor terminal plate is the connection point between nerve and muscle.

Motor neuron fibers conduct electrical impulses to the muscle cells to stimulate contractions.

Myofibrils are the components of muscle fiber

The actin filaments have a spiral form that couples them to the adjacent filaments of myosin to produce muscle contractions.

important part of the muscle, and thanks to which movement is carried out. They are a functional unit of the muscle in which the transformation of chemical energy into mechanical energy occurs. This is the process that causes muscle contractions.

THE NERVOUS SYSTEM

To better understand the effects of stretching, we must examine the nervous stimulation of the musculature.

This system is regulated by complex networks of nerves. These are very specialized, and they receive electrical signals originating from specific structures known as *receptors*, which are found on the inside of the muscles, directing the signals towards the CNS. These signals travel up the length of the spinal cord and arrive at the brain. En route, they unite with other signals originating from the rest of the skeletal muscle apparatus—these carry the

information arriving from the sense organs and those involved with the visceral system. Within the brain, these signals are integrated with information that derives from motor memory, cognitive memory, and emotional memory. Each gesture, action, movement, and sensation is stored in an archive in the brain from which we continually obtain data—e.g., to avoid injuring oneself with fire—without forgetting those skills and experiences we have learned in the past.

It is easy to intuit how highly specialized this system is: it is capable of originating impulses that go from the cranium through the specific nervous systemways (pyramidal and extrapyramidal) across a particular point (e.g., a motor neuron by the anterior horn of the spinal cord). From there it emits a final message or signal that traverses the motor plate, determining the response of the individual muscle—provoking *muscle contraction* or *release*.

Though on the face of it a very compli-

The motor cortex controls the voluntary muscle system. In the diagram at left, the brain's left hemisphere is in red, and in blue, the right (seen from behind). Nerve impulses from the cortex (1) pass through the brain stem via bundles of fibers that criss-cross at the juncture where the spinal column begins (2). The source of the nerve impulses is the right side of the brain, which controls the left side of the body and vice versa. These nerve impulses then pass from the medulla oblongata to fibers that cross the spinal stem (3), at which point they diverge and connect up with other neural appendages (4), such as the motor spinal cord roots (5), forming the spinal nerves (6) that finally transmit impulses to the effector muscles. The movements of the involuntary muscles are controlled by the fibers of the autonomic nervous system (seen in green), which pass from the motor spinal root to a chain adjacent to the nerve ganglia (7).

cated process and one not easily understood, it is in reality a very simple and mechanical one that is going on within us at every moment. Even now, as you are reading this book, this operation is made possible thanks to millions of neurons—muscle and nerve fibers whose constant collaboration permit us to create, change, and define the various positions of our body.

The techniques of stretching play a part in this process, creating a sense of equilibrium and bodily awareness that will prove useful in the sports field or in everyday life.

STRETCHING AND MUSCLES

What occurs at the muscular level during stretching? We have already seen that the motor neuron situated at the anterior horn of the spinal cord marks the point at which signals for muscle contraction begin to be sent. These must then pass through nerve circuits, which either facilitate or inhibit their activity and which screen out any movement that would damage the muscle structure.

Any activity, even one normally considered outside the ambit of athletic activities, can use stretching as an aid to further development.

The nervous stimulus is transmitted to the fibers by means both chemical and electric. When this stimulus, similar to an electric shock, reaches the motor plate, a chemical substance is released (called an acetylcholine) that starts an electric current flowing which, when it attains a certain intensity, triggers the (muscle) contraction. There exist in the muscle various specialized receptors that send messages in regard to its function—these now begin to help us to understand what is happening during a stretching exercise. Such receptors are as follows: the neuromuscular spindles, the Golgi tendon organs, and the nerve endings.

▶ The **neuromuscular spindles** are receptors typical of the striated voluntary muscle type. Each neuromuscular spindle is formed by a sheaf of muscular fibers and is separated from the rest of the muscle by a sheath. The function of the muscular spindles is that of adjusting muscle length, or rather, the difference in fiber length between the inner and outer spindles, making modifications as required.

Spindle activity can be of three kinds:

—Contractile: with the muscle at rest, the intrafusal fibers stretch, with the effect that contractions of the muscle also are eased (muscle tone);

—Stretching: a muscle that is stretched uses the central part of the neuromuscular spindle, responding reflexively, as the muscle springs back to its preceding length. The muscle will respond, lengthening and contracting accordingly, with the same intensity and speed as that applied to it;

—Shortening: during active muscle contraction, the spindle relaxes, a process that results in muscle shortening, in which position the muscle fibers are parallel.

One of the first rules to observe when becoming more acquainted with the practice of stretching is that of never trying to force any movement: Excessive strain can turn out to be painful or even harmful to the musculature.

IF IT CAUSES PAIN, THERE WILL BE NO GAIN

Assume a standing position, and with your arms at their sides, try to lower yourself slowly to the ground, keeping your legs straight; then try touching the floor with your hands. Now try to get even closer to the ground with your hands, helping yourself along with small movements. You will notice that after five or six such attempts, your hands move progressively closer to the ground. However, if after a minute you attempt to carry out this same exercise without those small movements, your hands will not even reach to where you were initially. This simple test is useful to show how the muscles can be worked excessively to their detriment. Not only does one risk microtraumas to the muscle fibers, but the strain will only give you opposite results. In other words, you must first warm up your muscles and prepare them for stretching.

With this simple and practical test, one can easily understand that the more the muscle is stretched and gets used to a certain kind of workout, the more evident will be the myofibrils' response to elongation. In fact, a defensive mechanism will come into play, giving way to a contraction (a reflex response to the muscle lengthening). If the muscle gets used to contracting rather than stretching, it will eventually lose the latter capacity. Advanced bodybuilding practices carry these concepts to the extreme, since an increase in muscle mass requires keeping these contractions going—usually without a pause during the entire exercise session.

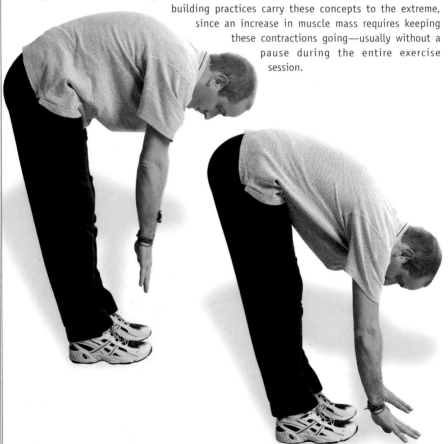

▶ The **Golgi tendon** organs and the free nerve endings help to control activity associated with muscle contraction; however, in regard to muscle elongation, they play another role that is just as important but difficult to state clearly in practical terms.

Put simply, these neural structures contain within them two specific mechanisms whose objective is that of opposing any excessive elongation that could damage the muscle texture. The first is called a reflex of distension and manifests itself as a certain muscle contraction, whose intensity is in direct proportion to the strain to which it is opposed. The second is defined as autogenic inhibition or an elongation reaction, which responds to excessive elongation by relaxing the muscle.

Such protective mechanisms intervene in predictable ways. When pulled suddenly, the muscle tends to react with a contraction; if this isn't sufficient, a second mechanism comes into play that allows the muscle to relax and consequently elongate.

The human muscular system defends itself from faults of posture using the muscular mechanisms that we have just described. This fact is verifiable with the simple and practical tests given earlier.

Never take an instance of pain to be a sign of success. While performing an exercise, allow yourself to be guided and stimulated by positive sensations, not painful ones.

The balance achieved between an exercise and the feelings derived from performing it must serve as the essential starting point for every individual who works out.

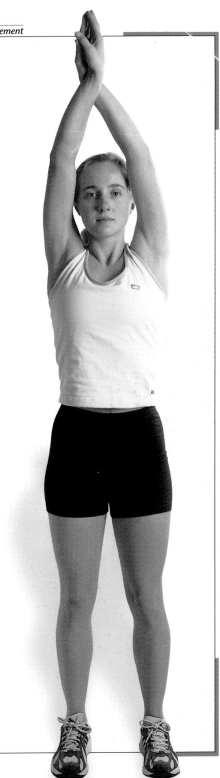

Why Stretch?

STRETCHING TECHNIQUES

The principal methodologies that apply to stretching can be reduced to two fundamental types: the connective tissue stretching of Bob Anderson and the tendonal (or dynamic) stretching of Sven Sölveborn.

These two types differ markedly in regard to difficulty of execution. Bob Anderson was an American trainer who in 1968 began to elaborate his method and assemble its core techniques. He taught them to various professional teams in the United States. The techniques are based on research, from which developed a progressive method of elongating the muscles. His method begins with simple tension as a means of arriving at a state of developed muscle tone.

The second method was researched and developed by Sven Sölveborn, a specialist in orthopedic surgery, a handball aficionado, and a high-level athletic trainer and member of the Swedish Society of Sports Medicine.

Motives for Stretching

Once the practice of stretching becomes a daily habit, it allows one to obtain, among other benefits, the following:

—Muscle relaxation and general stress relief.
—Improved posture and the ability to maintain it over the long term.
—Improved performance in sports activities.
—The capacity to "listen to your body" and interpret what it's saying to you.
—Better neuromuscular coordination.
—Increased blood flow and resultant lessening of injury risk.
—Pain relief, especially on or near the spinal column.
—The capacity to control one's breathing and to use the breathing apparatus in a more economical, efficient way.
—An improvement in one's sex life, thanks to the body's being more flexible and relaxed.

It is more advanced and is based on alternately contracting, relaxing, and elongating the muscles to obtain the best results.

Our text follows the method of Bob Anderson, as the latter has an easier application and is more widely known, both in the sporting sphere and at the personal-training level. However, for accurate information, and to improve one's store of knowledge, when discussing the exercises we will supply examples of Sölveborn's technique as well.

Overall we will present new forms of stretching that will be integrated into workouts, which deal either with the movement centers or with physical rehabilitation, in other words, relating to Proprioceptive Neuromuscular Facilitation, or PNF (see pages 80–81).

WORKOUT METHODS

To start, one should always keep in mind the following basic concept: the suggestions given herein do not

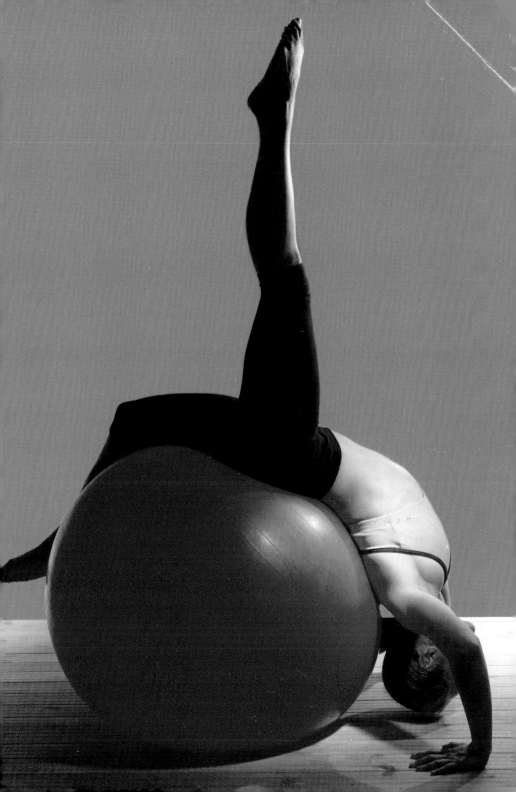

represent a fixed way of doing things; rather, we are offering general guidelines. Since the attributes and fitness level of each person vary, we will take this as a fundamental point of departure.

To obtain good results, it is important to undertake at least three 15-minute exercise sessions per week or, if possible, to work out once daily. In this way, one can create a daily habit that will eventually become second nature.

THE PART BREATHING PLAYS IN EXERCISE

As already noted, one of the principal aims of stretching is that of helping the body to maintain, and in most cases, to recover, the capacity for relaxation. To do this, it is of fundamental importance to know how to control the breathing process.

Therefore, let us expand further on this important principle. Each time a person gets ready to carry out a new movement—especially in dealing with the first steps, and even more so when one is reentering sports after a hiatus—a full complement of muscles will be used, including those that are not directly related to the activity the person is focusing attention on. Instinctively, each person will adjust his movement so as to make it as precise as possible. For example, when confronting any new type of movement, one will draw on one's motor memory in order to respond to a new request from the brain; through repeated trial and error, one reaches the point where one has perfected the new movement. Such a learning process brings into play the entire body, which acquires new knowledge through successive stages of exercise. In all this, respiration plays a key role.

▶ Respiration comprises two phases: *inhalation* and *exhalation*. The first is the active phase, and is characterized by the contraction of the diaphragm and its surrounding muscles. The second is the passive phase, during which the diaphragm and the muscles involved relax, permitting the rib cage to return to a state of rest. Breathing also involves the rest of the muscles: during inhalation, the spinal column extends itself, whereas during exhalation, it returns to a rest state.

We now present an example that will elucidate this point: if you are seated in a very comfortable position, it is possible to inhale deeply through the nose in order to fill the lungs to their maximum capacity. You will notice that your chest will be thrust forward and consequently, your head will be held higher and your posture be more erect.

To help us understand the relationship between relaxation and exhalation, we can look at the similar relationship that exists between the cardiac and respiratory systems. While inhaling, we are able to feel our heartbeat accelerating, whereas when we exhale, our heart rate tends to decrease. At the same time, the body's activities, both sympathetic and parasympathetic (i.e., the autonomic nervous system) fluctuate. This phenomenon explains why respiratory control is fundamental to inducing relaxation during numerous activities.

Based on the foregoing, we can say that the main working principle of stretching involves allowing the muscles to relax; coupled with control of respiration, we achieve the desired results.

Moving about in free and open spaces can make physical activity more pleasant and relaxing. Your respiration will improve, and you will receive positive reinforcement for your daily workouts.

▶ It is important to breathe slowly and in a relaxed manner, and to try exhaling while a muscle is being stretched. The best way to breathe is to inhale through the nose while expanding the abdomen during the movement of the diaphragm. Hold the air inside your lungs for a moment, and then exhale slowly through the nose or mouth. It is advisable to practice inhaling through the nose, because in this way the inhaled air is filtered, warmed, and moistened.

Breathing from the diaphragm should not require great exertion, but should be a natural process of contraction and relaxation. During inhalation, the diaphragm pushes downward toward the internal organs and their surrounding structures. The blood is pumped out of the vessels, and when you exhale, the organs within the abdomen receive oxygen-rich blood.

The rhythmic movements of the diaphragm permit the lungs to carry out the needed exchange of oxygen for carbon dioxide. They also improve the circulation, which in turn speeds up the process of eliminating waste products (e.g., lactic acid and other metabolites) that build up in the system as a result of muscle activity.

STRETCHING AND EATING HABITS

Performing stretching exercises under extreme conditions, such as fasting or overeating, is misguided and counterproductive. The following is not intended as a treatise on diet; however, it will help you to become acquainted, as closely as possible, with what constitutes a balanced diet. This practice should enter your daily routine, along with your commitment to regular stretching.

A balanced diet includes a wide variety of foods that provide the body with the necessary energy to grow and repair itself. In order to survive, we need the following nutrients:
—Proteins (found in fish, eggs, cereals, whole grains, nut products, beans, dried fruit, and meat) that furnish 4,000 calories
—Fats (found, for example, in cheeses, butter, and olive oil) that furnish 9,000 calories
—Carbohydrates (found in bread, pasta, potatoes, rice, and grains) that furnish 4,000 calories
—Vitamins (fat-soluble vitamins A, D, E, and K, which are found in cheese and fish; and water-soluble vitamins C and B, which are found in green vegetables and fruits).
—Minerals (e.g., calcium, potassium, sulfur, phosphorous, sodium, magnesium, and chloride, which are found in cauliflower, spinach, lettuce, and lentils).

In addition to this list, we must include dietary fiber (found in fruits, vegetables, and whole-grain breads) and, most importantly, water.

The nutrition pyramid indicates, how much attention should be paid to various elements of nutrition.

Energy Requirements

To understand the foundation of a balanced diet, it is first necessary to explain what is meant by energy requirements. The quantity of energy necessary for an organism can be divided into two parts: that which is necessary to maintain basal metabolism (i.e., minimal energy for an organism at rest, either physically or psychologically), and that which allows one to undertake an activity. Energy requirements vary according to age, sex, physical constitution, overall health, and the activity being performed; these requirements are heightened in particular situations, such as pregnancy, breastfeeding, and menopause.

Energy from food intake should be derived from the following sources:
—60% carbohydrates
—30% fats
—10% proteins
Based on this distribution, the food pyramid offers clear guidance for nutrition in your daily life.

PHYSICAL CONDITION AND STRETCHING

Stretching is an activity that does not carry particular risks, and for this reason is adaptable to individuals of any age and sex. However, before taking on the work and determining your physical state, some suggestions should be taken into consideration.

Pay close attention to developing exercises that tend to isolate specific regions of the body.

Such exercises help us to prevent reawakening painful symptoms that can result from the following medical conditions: problems of the spinal column (e.g., herniated disks, fractured vertebrae); problems of the knee ligaments (loose ligaments, torn ligaments, postoperative damage); and problems of the muscles (e.g., pulls or tears). Be mindful of these potential problems in relation to the exercises that will be suggested further on.

During periods of illness (e.g., flu), it is best to limit or even take a break from physical work until fully regaining your health. But pay attention—don't let the "symptoms" of laziness interfere with your ongoing commitment to getting into better physical shape.

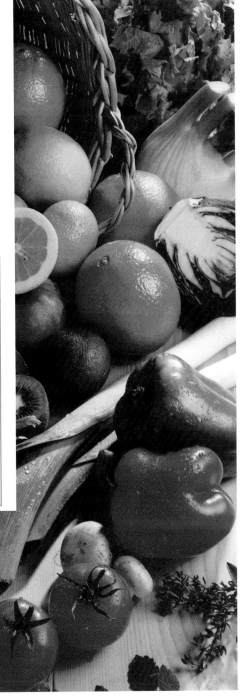

Eating In and Working Out

It is important to remember:
—Do not exercise right after you have eaten because the digestive system will not function optimally;
—Do not exercise right before mealtime, or if you feel hungry, because your appetite will interfere with your concentration;
—Before an exercise session—especially if you plan to eat lunch or dinner many hours later—it is advisable to eat a fruit or something else that is easily digestible.

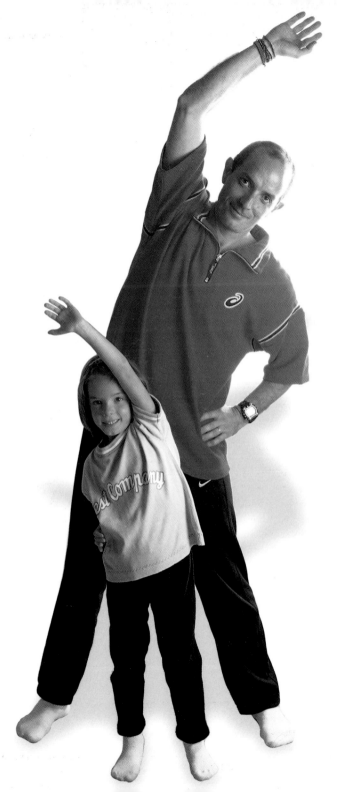

Gymnastic stretching may be practiced at many age levels and for a variety of reasons; it can also be enriching if practiced in a social setting.

Stretching Out

Some fundamental guidelines for stretching are listed below. Follow these rules to develop a safe and effective exercise regimen.

PREPARING TO EXERCISE

As it has been important to establish certain basic concepts leading up to the stretching exercises, it is also important to know how to prepare your body for stretching. This phase of the workout is called the warm-up.

Warming up allows the least experienced person to organize the workout session more effectively. Warming up guarantees that you will achieve the best result from the exercises that follow. Warm-ups offer:

—Improved muscle control and elasticity;
—Respiratory and cardiovascular system efficiency;
—Heightened knowledge and awareness of sensations that arise during a workout.

The activity of warming up can be subdivided into two phases: joint movement (isolation exercises) and aerobic activity.

THE ELEMENTS OF A GOOD STRETCH

Getting positive results from a stretching workout depends on several factors: isolating the muscles, assuming various positions, and setting the duration of the exercises.

Muscle Isolation

To work out effectively, it is fundamental to use only the targeted muscles without involving neighboring muscle structures. Try not to activate opposing muscles that will interfere with the movement you are performing; in sum, the fewer muscles that are included in a movement, the better the specific muscle, or small group of muscles, will be able to stretch out. When you isolate a muscle that should be stretched, you have more control, and consequently, the possibility of var-ying the intensity of the exercise. This leads to progressively better results.

Important Tips for Stretching

Don't forget these fundamental ground rules for correct execution:
—Never accept pain as normal;
—Respect your limits, but don't underestimate your potential;
—Try to work up to the stretches slowly and progressively;
—Never bounce up and down during the exercises—doing so may cause cramps or internal injury;
—Do not use weights.

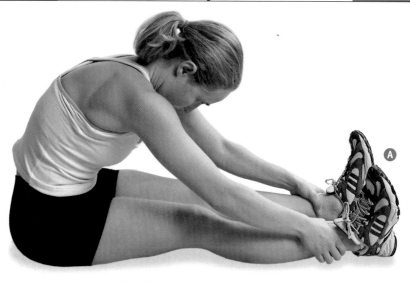

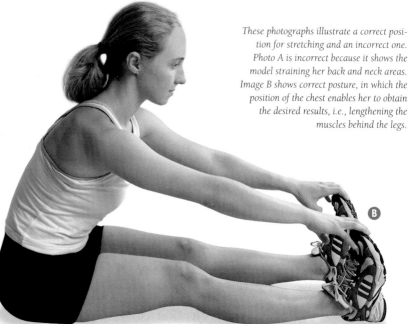

These photographs illustrate a correct position for stretching and an incorrect one. Photo A is incorrect because it shows the model straining her back and neck areas. Image B shows correct posture, in which the position of the chest enables her to obtain the desired results, i.e., lengthening the muscles behind the legs.

Positions

If the positions are maintained correctly, as indicated, the exercises will be more efficient. In addition, you will gain greater control over their intensity without having to use more force. If you find yourself in an incorrect position, you always run the risk of harming your muscle structures and ligaments. The exercises will become more effective and simple if you assume positions that are under your conscious direction.

Exercise Duration

There are no precise laws that regulate how long you should maintain the various stretching positions. However, there are diverse theories proposing various times—anywhere from 10 seconds to 2–3 minutes, or alternatively, 30 seconds to 1 minute. Other experts still (certainly creating more confusion) believe that 15 seconds is the maximum time to stretch for lengthening and maintaining tendon structures while, in total contradiction, affirming that 15 seconds is not sufficient for muscle elongation. One thing that is certain, however, is that children and adolescents, whose bones are still developing, should stretch for around 7–10 seconds in each position to avoid hindering their growth process too much.

To summarize, we give the following general recommendations:

—7–10 seconds is the duration for holding each position by growing children and adolescents.

—20–30 seconds is the advisable time for adults to hold positions to eliminate tension and attain true flexibility.

As already stated, our directions refer to the method utilized by the largest percentage of people who practice sports, and which is, most importantly, easier to perform: the method of Bob Anderson.

Easy and Advanced Stretching

In approaching Anderson's method, two fundamental, related concepts have to be clarified: they relate to **simple tension** and **conditioning tension**.

Relaxed stretching uses simple tension and is maintained without bouncing, while breathing regularly, and releasing the stretch at 15- to 25-second intervals. Its goal is to prepare the muscle tissue for the next round of conditioning, and above all, to protect the opposing muscles from strain. The feeling of tension should diminish while performing the exercises. If it does not, you will need to loosen the muscle until the tension stops.

With regard to conditioning tension, it should be easily maintained for 10–20 seconds longer than the simple tension exercises. You maintain the same position as you do for simple tension stretching, while trying to increase the sensation that you feel on the muscular level. As in the preceding, this type of stretching exercise must be carried out with relaxed breathing, and should lower your body's overall stress level. It should give you a feeling of greater healthfulness and heightened sensitivity.

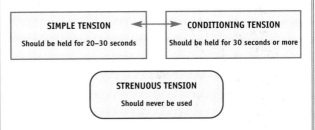

SIMPLE TENSION	CONDITIONING TENSION
Should be held for 20–30 seconds	Should be held for 30 seconds or more

STRENUOUS TENSION
Should never be used

Strenuous tension results when you ignore the two previous phases and their accompanying muscle sensations. This type of tension is accompanied by severe pain and a pressing need to change positions. Although many people believe that stretching is all about "no pain, no gain," as we have seen, this idea is absolutely incorrect.

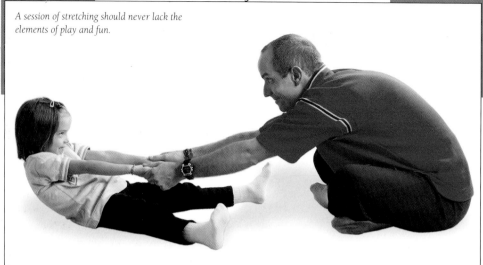

A session of stretching should never lack the elements of play and fun.

WHEN TO PERFORM THE EXERCISES

It may seem boring and repetitive, but the best time to perform these exercises always depends on the condition and preparation of the muscles. To put it more simply, it depends on whether they are already "warmed up" thanks to the activities discussed earlier.

With regard to time of day, there is no precise and fixed rule for when to stretch. However, it is important to establish a regular routine. Many people tend to follow their own internal biological clock, "knowing" which moment of the day is optimal for stretching. Some feel a great burst of energy and are predisposed to exercise in the morning, whereas others are so inclined during the afternoon or evening.

From the statistical point of view, one notes that a good number of people are more mobile and flexible in the afternoon than in the morning, achieving a maximum ability at around 2:30 p.m. to 4:00 p.m. as well as in the later hours.

If, however, for personal reasons and especially for time management, you should use a wristwatch, along with your biological clock, to decide when to exercise, it is important to do this in such a way that the exercises will be carried out with attention. Keep in mind that muscles are usually less elastic and flexible at night; even when adhering to a set schedule, it is advisable to listen to your body and respect its needs.

CLOTHING

While working out, extremely comfortable clothes that permit freedom of movement are indispensable. It is essential to take off accessories (e.g., necklaces, ties, belts) that limit your ability to move.

Nevertheless, the environment or the particular situation may not allow you to change clothes, e.g., at the office during work, or in some brief pause in your busy daily routine. If so, you can remain dressed the way you are, perhaps just loosening your belt or tie, or opening a button of your skirt or pants in order to perform some simple movements with the least constraint.

Warming Up

Step 1: Joint Mobility Exercises

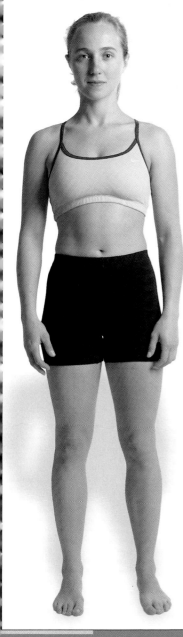

Exercising individual joints allows you to improve their lubrication during stretching by involving the *synovial fluid*. This fluid prepares the joint to deal with the work of stretching, but above all, it allows you to practice the physical activity or sport that interests you most.

These preparatory exercises are effective owing to their slow, circular movements, both clockwise and counterclockwise. They never require the joints to become overextended, and therefore do not overwork or put unnecessary strain on the body.

The order of the following exercises makes for a logical progression, beginning with the tips of the toes and ending with the top of the head. They involve all parts of the body, namely:

•Toes •Ankles
•Knees •Hips
•The lumbar region (lower-back region),
•The dorsal region (upper body)
•Shoulders
•Elbows •Hands
•Head and neck

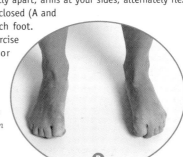

Toes

▸ **EXERCISE 1**
Standing, legs slightly apart, arms at your sides, alternately flex your toes open and closed (A and B), 10 times for each foot. You may do this exercise with shoes on or barefoot.

Warming up your toes improves their function and general health, along with that of the entire body.

Ankles

▶ **EXERCISE 2**

Standing, with legs slightly apart, arms at your sides, rotate your right foot in one direction and then in the other. Perform the same motions with your left foot, repeating them 10 times for each foot.

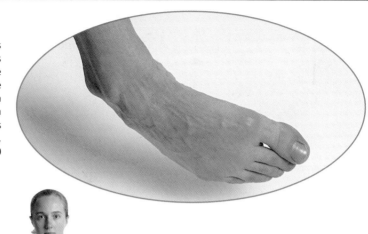

Extending your arms to the sides helps you maintain your balance during this exercise.

Ⓐ

Knees

▶ **EXERCISE 3**

Standing, with legs slightly apart and arms extended to each side (A), raise your right leg with your knee slightly bent; then swing your lower leg from the knee, forward and back. Repeat this movement with the left foot (B) for a total of 10 times per foot.

Ⓑ

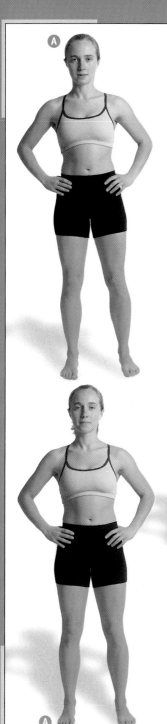

Hips

▶ **EXERCISE 4**

Stand with your legs slightly open, hands on your hips (A). Twist your right leg, from the foot to the top of the thigh, first toward your right and then toward your left (B). Repeat this movement with the left leg for a total of 10 times per leg.

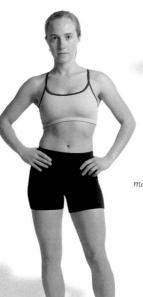

To successfully perform this exercise, it is important not to move your shoulders at any time.

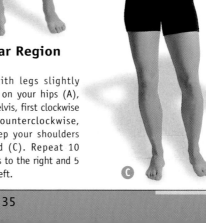

Lumbar Region

▶ **EXERCISE 5**

Standing, with legs slightly apart, hands on your hips (A), rotate your pelvis, first clockwise and then counterclockwise, trying to keep your shoulders still (B) and (C). Repeat 10 times: 5 times to the right and 5 times to the left.

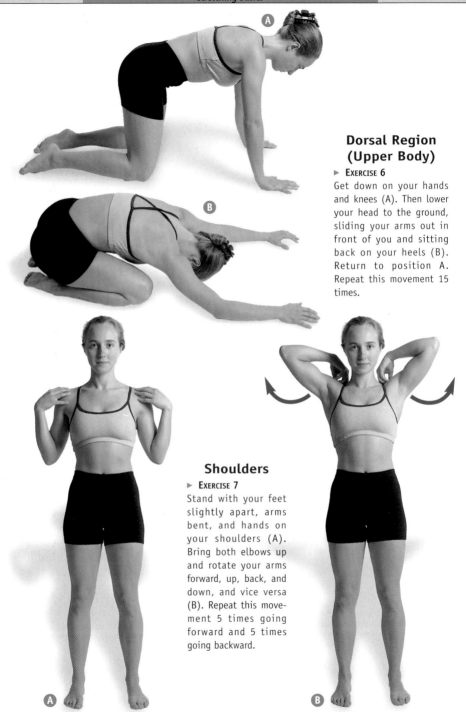

Dorsal Region (Upper Body)

▶ EXERCISE 6

Get down on your hands and knees (A). Then lower your head to the ground, sliding your arms out in front of you and sitting back on your heels (B). Return to position A. Repeat this movement 15 times.

Shoulders

▶ EXERCISE 7

Stand with your feet slightly apart, arms bent, and hands on your shoulders (A). Bring both elbows up and rotate your arms forward, up, back, and down, and vice versa (B). Repeat this movement 5 times going forward and 5 times going backward.

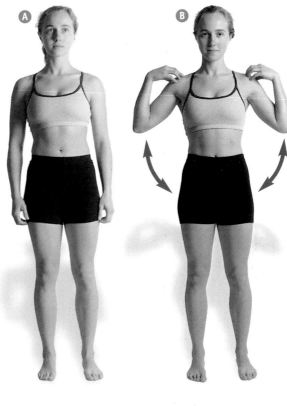

Elbows

▶ **EXERCISE 8**
Stand with your feet slightly apart, arms bent, and hands at your sides (A). Bring your hands simultaneously up to touch your shoulders and back down again. Repeat 10 times.

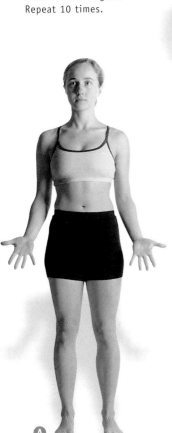

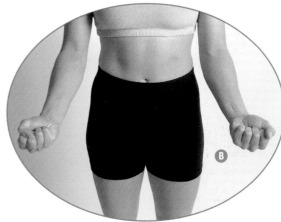

Hands

▶ **EXERCISE 9**
Stand with your feet slightly apart and arms bent outward. Fully open and close your fingers 10 times (A and B).

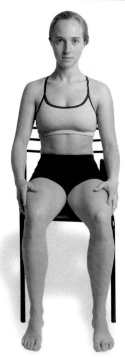

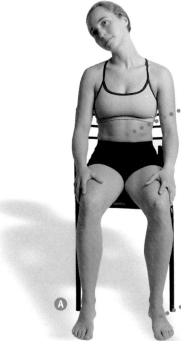

Use your abdominal muscles to support your back's lumbar region, which touches the chair back.

Try to maintain this back support by keeping the soles of your feet against the floor.

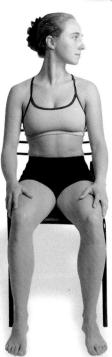

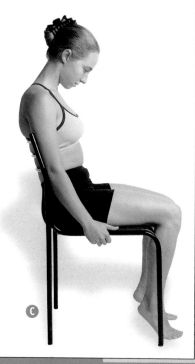

Head and Neck

▶ **EXERCISE 10**

Sit with your back supported against a wall and your legs crossed, or sit in a chair with back support.

Tilt your head to the right and to the left 6 times (A).

Turn your head to the right and to the left 6 times (B).

Bend your head forward and raise it up 6 times (C).

Step 2: Aerobic Activity

After you have performed the joint-mobility exercises, it is time to do some aerobic work that is not strenuous. It should continue for 3 to 4 minutes, in order to stimulate the cardiovascular system and circulation and to increase your heart rate and respiration. The goal of this activity is to improve blood flow to the muscles and, as a consequence, to decrease the risk of harming the muscles. Aerobic activities include running outdoors or in place, jumping rope, or moving to the rhythm of music. During these exercises, try to notice the physiological changes taking place that were discussed above.

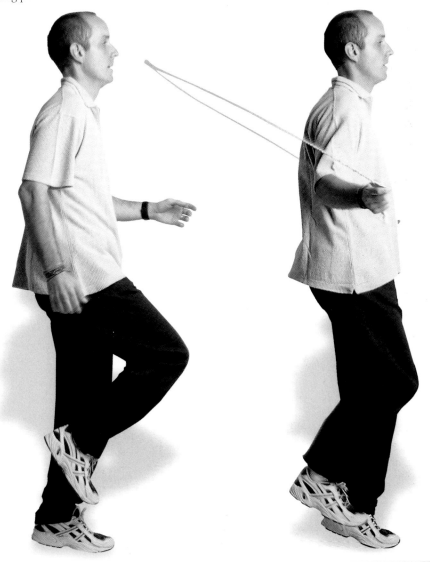

Step 3: Massage

Self-massage is a powerful treatment for the muscles, especially before stretching. Massaging the muscles confers the following benefits:

—Improved blood circulation to the muscles;

—Relaxation of the particular muscle that will be stretched;

—Removal of substances (waste products, e.g., lactic acid) that have accumulated after a physical workout.

The simplest method for performing self-massage is to imagine that you have a small piece of soap between your hands. You "apply" the soap to all parts of your body, manipulating and moving it with particular pressure and paying special attention to parts of the body that will be involved in stretching. If you have time, you may self-massage your entire body.

► **EXERCISE 1**
Sitting cross-legged and without shoes (A), grasp your left foot with your hands and using your thumbs, deeply massage the sole of your foot (B). Repeat the procedure with your other foot.

A

B

► **EXERCISE 2**
Still seated, place your hands on your right calf and massage the entire area. Do the same with the other calf.

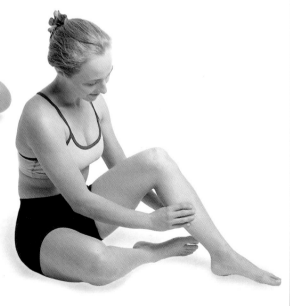

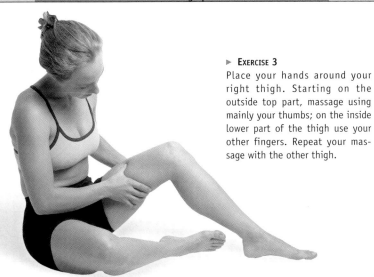

▶ **EXERCISE 3**
Place your hands around your right thigh. Starting on the outside top part, massage using mainly your thumbs; on the inside lower part of the thigh use your other fingers. Repeat your massage with the other thigh.

▶ **EXERCISE 4**
Place your palm on your abdomen. Starting with your navel, make a clockwise spiral movement until your fingers reach the border of your rib cage. Continue to circle until your fingers reach the pubic area. Repeat your spiral motion, starting from the rib cage and ending back at the center.

▶ **EXERCISE 5**
Using your thumbs as support, massage the lumbar region of your back, continuing up to the top.

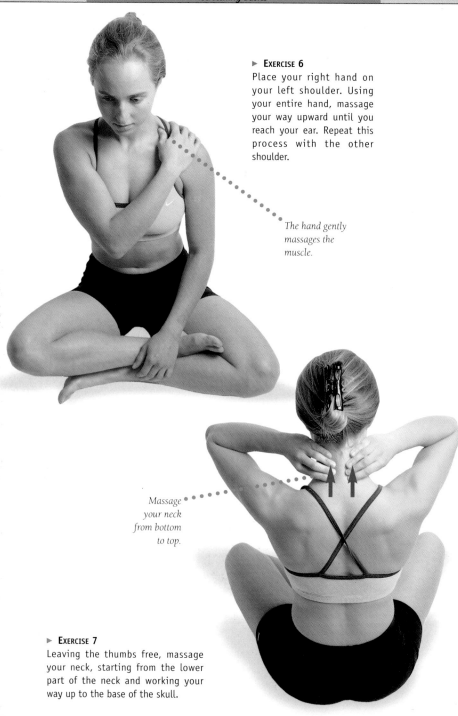

▶ **EXERCISE 6**
Place your right hand on your left shoulder. Using your entire hand, massage your way upward until you reach your ear. Repeat this process with the other shoulder.

The hand gently massages the muscle.

Massage your neck from bottom to top.

▶ **EXERCISE 7**
Leaving the thumbs free, massage your neck, starting from the lower part of the neck and working your way up to the base of the skull.

► **EXERCISE 8**
Massage your hands vigorously, as if washing them under running water.

The massage begins at the wrist and ends at the shoulder.

► **EXERCISE 9**
With your left hand, massage your right wrist, working your way up toward the right shoulder. Vigorously massage the entire forearm, elbow, upper arm, and shoulders. Repeat with the left arm.

Stretching Exercises
According to Anderson

The following are the two criteria that determine the order of the exercises:
–Division into specific area of the body (feet, ankles, calves, etc.).
–Level of difficulty of execution (for each part of the body, we have indicated groups of exercises in order of increasing difficulty in respect to the muscle exertion required during the stretch).

To follow the instructions correctly, you will be shown the position, how to breathe, and how to hold the positions. Your results will be better insofar as you are consistent and regular in your workouts.

We do not explicitly indicate how much time is needed to maintain the positions presented; instead, each person should set the time and duration of the exercise according to his or her level of preparation, desire, and ability.

Feet

▶ **EXERCISE 1**
Sitting with your legs crossed, place your right leg over your left leg. Grasp your right foot with your left hand, sliding your fingers between your toes. Spread your toes apart until you reach the base of your fingers. Repeat with your other foot.

► **EXERCISE 2**

Sit with your legs crossed. Grasp the toes of your left foot in your right hand; using your hand, curl your toes up, towards you (A). Then extend them outward, towards the floor (B). Repeat this exercise with the other foot.

► **EXERCISE 3**

While standing, lean against a wall, supported with one hand. Curl your toes in, against the floor. Starting with your big toe, roll your foot to the side, finishing with the small toe (A and B). Try to press the top of your foot towards the floor. Repeat with other the foot.

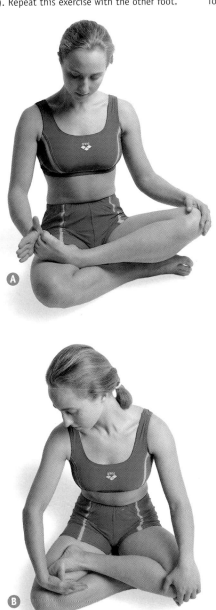

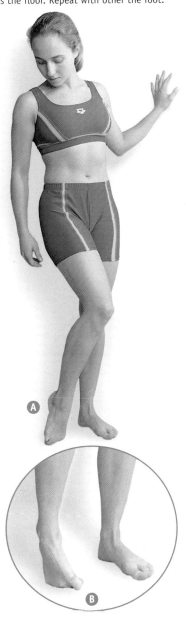

Ankles

▶ **EXERCISE 1**

Sit with your right leg extended in front of you and your left leg crossed over the top of your right thigh. While trying to leave the foot completely relaxed, rotate it in one direction and then the other (A). Repeat this movement with your other foot.

Without applying too much pressure, concentrate on the way your ankle moves.

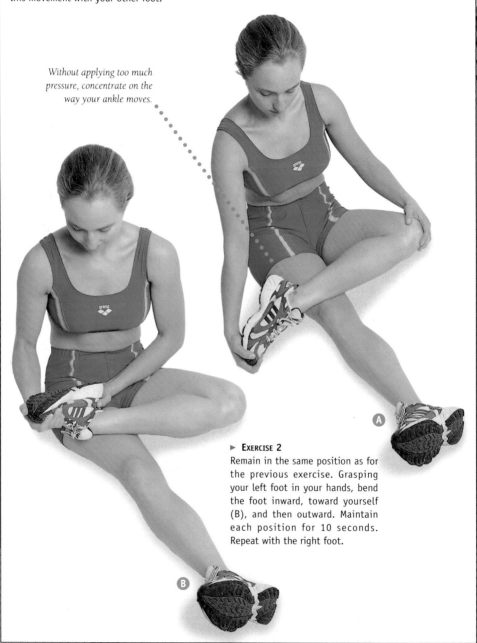

▶ **EXERCISE 2**

Remain in the same position as for the previous exercise. Grasping your left foot in your hands, bend the foot inward, toward yourself (B), and then outward. Maintain each position for 10 seconds. Repeat with the right foot.

► **EXERCISE 3**
Stand with your legs slightly apart, hands on your hips (A). Shift the weight of your body to the outside part of your feet (B) and then to the inside (C). Alternate the two positions, holding each of them.

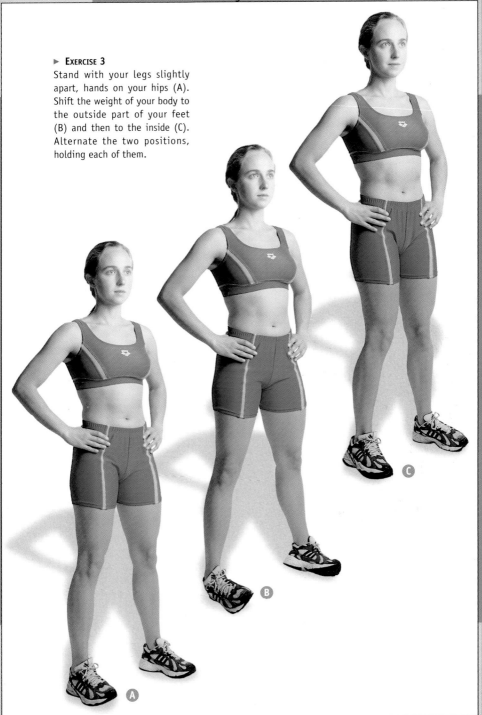

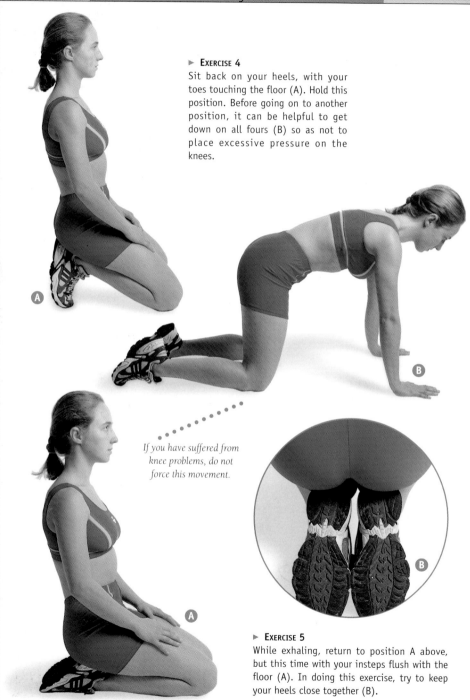

▶ **Exercise 4**

Sit back on your heels, with your toes touching the floor (A). Hold this position. Before going on to another position, it can be helpful to get down on all fours (B) so as not to place excessive pressure on the knees.

If you have suffered from knee problems, do not force this movement.

▶ **Exercise 5**

While exhaling, return to position A above, but this time with your insteps flush with the floor (A). In doing this exercise, try to keep your heels close together (B).

Calves

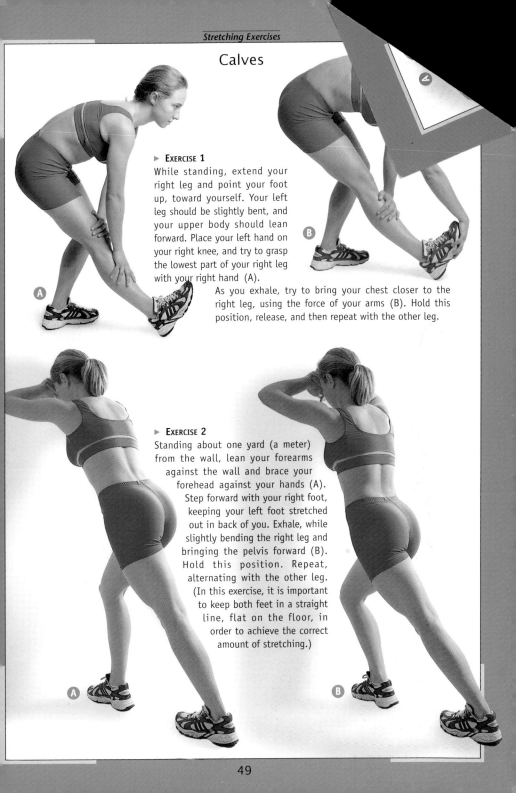

► **EXERCISE 1**

While standing, extend your right leg and point your foot up, toward yourself. Your left leg should be slightly bent, and your upper body should lean forward. Place your left hand on your right knee, and try to grasp the lowest part of your right leg with your right hand (A).

As you exhale, try to bring your chest closer to the right leg, using the force of your arms (B). Hold this position, release, and then repeat with the other leg.

► **EXERCISE 2**

Standing about one yard (a meter) from the wall, lean your forearms against the wall and brace your forehead against your hands (A). Step forward with your right foot, keeping your left foot stretched out in back of you. Exhale, while slightly bending the right leg and bringing the pelvis forward (B). Hold this position. Repeat, alternating with the other leg. (In this exercise, it is important to keep both feet in a straight line, flat on the floor, in order to achieve the correct amount of stretching.)

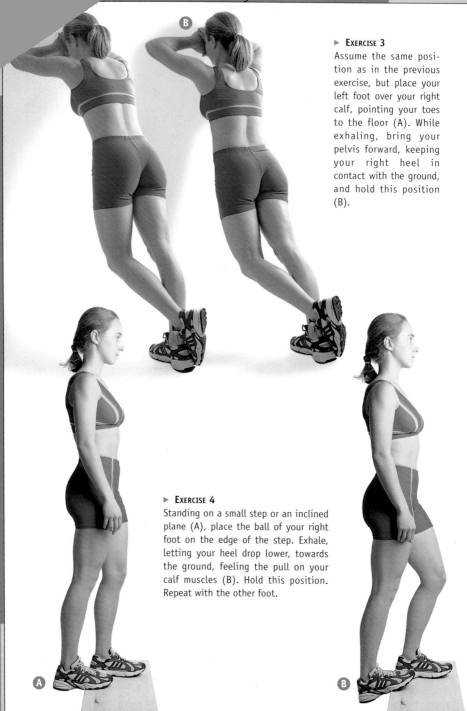

► **EXERCISE 3**
Assume the same position as in the previous exercise, but place your left foot over your right calf, pointing your toes to the floor (A). While exhaling, bring your pelvis forward, keeping your right heel in contact with the ground, and hold this position (B).

► **EXERCISE 4**
Standing on a small step or an inclined plane (A), place the ball of your right foot on the edge of the step. Exhale, letting your heel drop lower, towards the ground, feeling the pull on your calf muscles (B). Hold this position. Repeat with the other foot.

Abductor Muscles of the Thigh

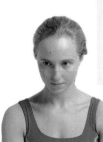

▶ **EXERCISE 1**
Sit on the floor with your feet together, legs bent out to the sides (A). Grasp the tops of your feet. While exhaling, press your knees down to the floor, holding the latter position (B). Relax and repeat.

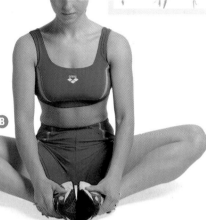

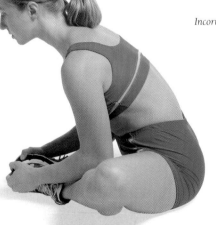

▶ **EXERCISE 2**
In the same position as the preceding, exhale, slowing bringing your navel area slowly towards the ground. Hold this position, relax, and repeat. In this movement, you must control the position of the upper body, which should be held erect during the bending.

Incorrect! • • • • • • • • • • •

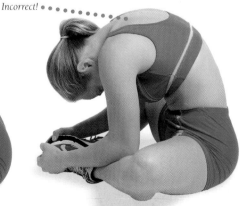

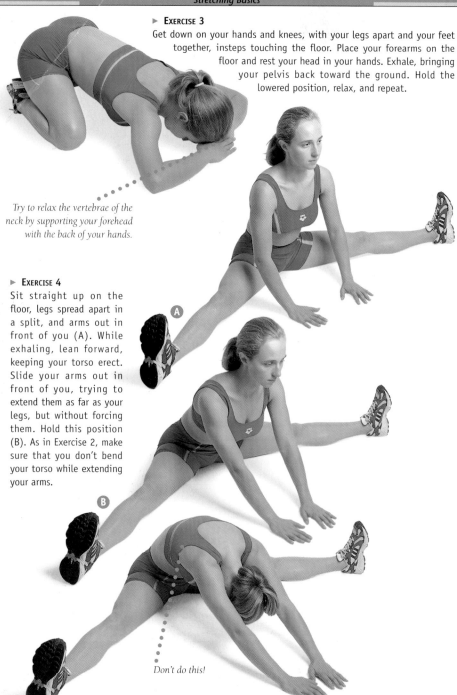

► EXERCISE 3

Get down on your hands and knees, with your legs apart and your feet together, insteps touching the floor. Place your forearms on the floor and rest your head in your hands. Exhale, bringing your pelvis back toward the ground. Hold the lowered position, relax, and repeat.

Try to relax the vertebrae of the neck by supporting your forehead with the back of your hands.

► EXERCISE 4

Sit straight up on the floor, legs spread apart in a split, and arms out in front of you (A). While exhaling, lean forward, keeping your torso erect. Slide your arms out in front of you, trying to extend them as far as your legs, but without forcing them. Hold this position (B). As in Exercise 2, make sure that you don't bend your torso while extending your arms.

Ⓐ

Ⓑ

Don't do this!

Quadriceps

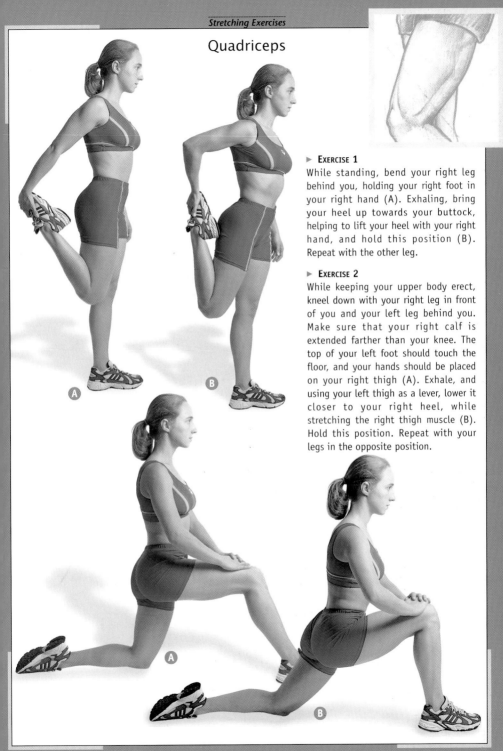

▶ **EXERCISE 1**

While standing, bend your right leg behind you, holding your right foot in your right hand (A). Exhaling, bring your heel up towards your buttock, helping to lift your heel with your right hand, and hold this position (B). Repeat with the other leg.

▶ **EXERCISE 2**

While keeping your upper body erect, kneel down with your right leg in front of you and your left leg behind you. Make sure that your right calf is extended farther than your knee. The top of your left foot should touch the floor, and your hands should be placed on your right thigh (A). Exhale, and using your left thigh as a lever, lower it closer to your right heel, while stretching the right thigh muscle (B). Hold this position. Repeat with your legs in the opposite position.

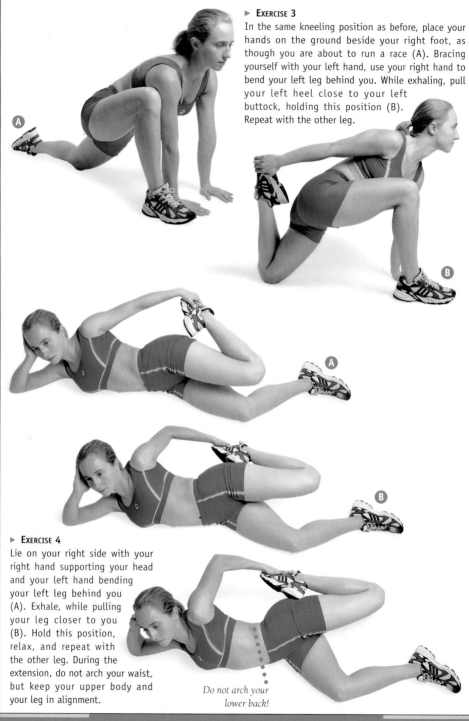

▶ **EXERCISE 3**

In the same kneeling position as before, place your hands on the ground beside your right foot, as though you are about to run a race (A). Bracing yourself with your left hand, use your right hand to bend your left leg behind you. While exhaling, pull your right heel close to your left buttock, holding this position (B). Repeat with the other leg.

▶ **EXERCISE 4**

Lie on your right side with your right hand supporting your head and your left hand bending your left leg behind you (A). Exhale, while pulling your leg closer to you (B). Hold this position, relax, and repeat with the other leg. During the extension, do not arch your waist, but keep your upper body and your leg in alignment.

Do not arch your lower back!

54

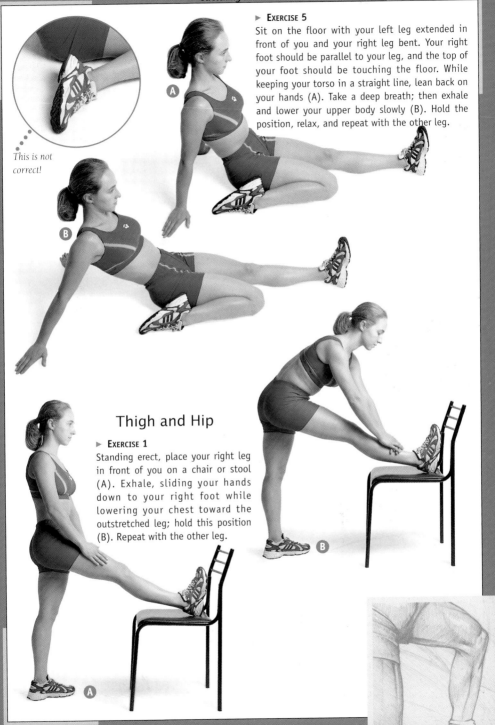

This is not correct!

▶ **Exercise 5**

Sit on the floor with your left leg extended in front of you and your right leg bent. Your right foot should be parallel to your leg, and the top of your foot should be touching the floor. While keeping your torso in a straight line, lean back on your hands (A). Take a deep breath; then exhale and lower your upper body slowly (B). Hold the position, relax, and repeat with the other leg.

Thigh and Hip

▶ **Exercise 1**

Standing erect, place your right leg in front of you on a chair or stool (A). Exhale, sliding your hands down to your right foot while lowering your chest toward the outstretched leg; hold this position (B). Repeat with the other leg.

► **EXERCISE 2**

Sitting with your right leg out in front of you and the left leg bent, place the sole of your foot on the inside of the right thigh. Grasp a rope or a piece of cord about a yard (one meter) long and loop the rope around your right foot (A). Exhale, wrapping the rope around your hands to tighten it while your navel area bends down, toward your extended leg. When you cannot move any closer, hold that position (B). Relax and repeat with the other foot. The chest must remain tilted—not hunched over—so as not to cause harm to the waist and lower back.

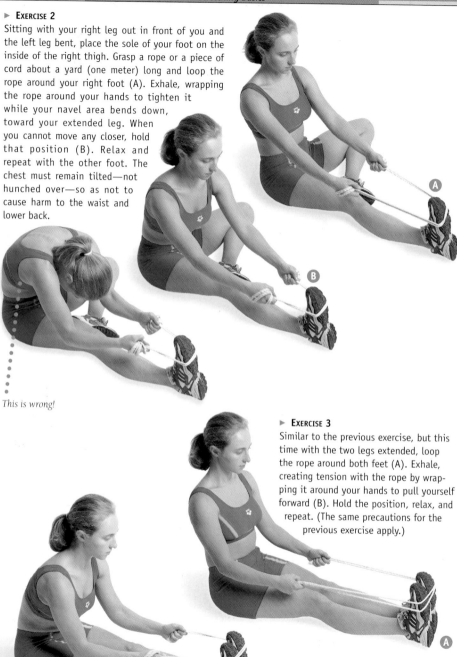

This is wrong!

► **EXERCISE 3**

Similar to the previous exercise, but this time with the two legs extended, loop the rope around both feet (A). Exhale, creating tension with the rope by wrapping it around your hands to pull yourself forward (B). Hold the position, relax, and repeat. (The same precautions for the previous exercise apply.)

▶ **EXERCISE 4**

Sit with your right leg extended straight out and your left leg bent, placing your left foot against the inside of your right thigh (A). While exhaling, bring your left hand toward your right foot and your right hand toward your left knee, passing your right arm through the space created between the right leg and the left arm (B). Hold the position, relax, and repeat with the other side.

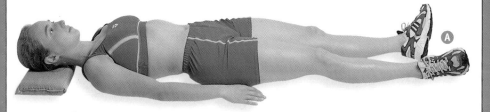

Gluteals

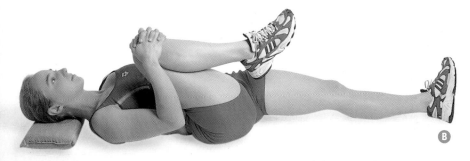

▶ **EXERCISE 1**

Lay down on your back (A). Bend your right leg up, grasping your knee between your hands. Now breathe out and pull the leg closer to your chest with your arms (B). Hold the position. Relax and repeat with the other leg.

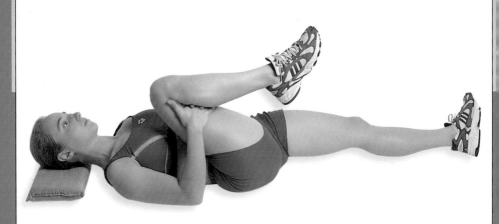

▶ **EXERCISE 2**

Position yourself as in the preceding exercise, but grasp the back of your thigh behind your knee. Exhale, drawing your leg towards the chest. Hold the position, relax, and repeat with the other leg.

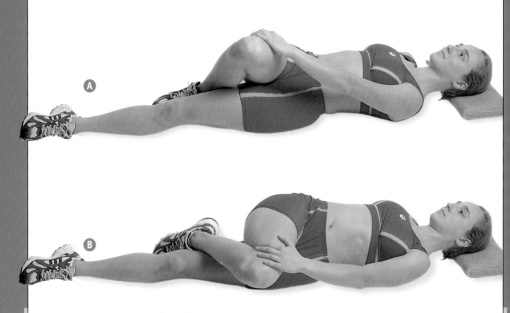

▶ **EXERCISE 3**

Lie on the ground with your left foot turned outward and your right leg bent over your left thigh. Place your left hand on top of the right thigh and exhale (A), slowly pushing your right leg over the left thigh and holding the position (B). Relax and repeat with the other leg.

Lower Back—Lumbar Zone

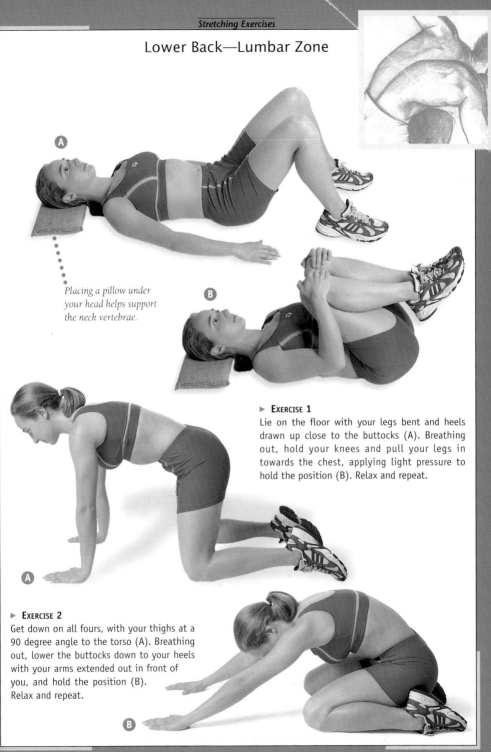

Placing a pillow under your head helps support the neck vertebrae.

▶ **EXERCISE 1**
Lie on the floor with your legs bent and heels drawn up close to the buttocks (A). Breathing out, hold your knees and pull your legs in towards the chest, applying light pressure to hold the position (B). Relax and repeat.

▶ **EXERCISE 2**
Get down on all fours, with your thighs at a 90 degree angle to the torso (A). Breathing out, lower the buttocks down to your heels with your arms extended out in front of you, and hold the position (B). Relax and repeat.

► **EXERCISE 3**

Lie on the floor with your legs bent and heels drawn up close to your buttocks (A). Exhale, pushing your pelvis in and down, thereby flattening the curve of the waist (B). Hold the position and repeat.

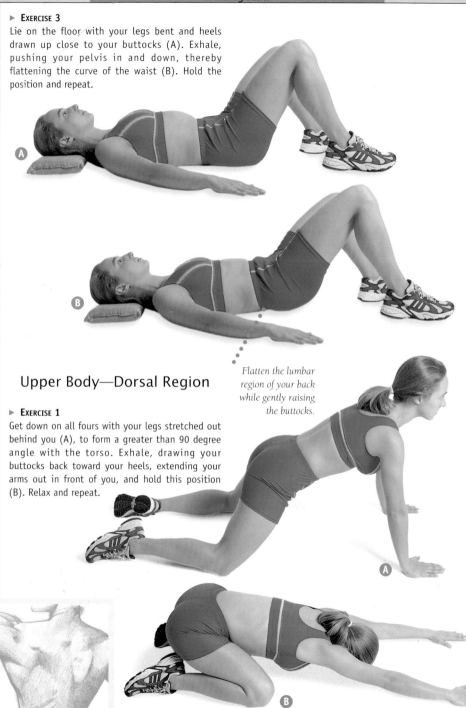

Upper Body—Dorsal Region

Flatten the lumbar region of your back while gently raising the buttocks.

► **EXERCISE 1**

Get down on all fours with your legs stretched out behind you (A), to form a greater than 90 degree angle with the torso. Exhale, drawing your buttocks back toward your heels, extending your arms out in front of you, and hold this position (B). Relax and repeat.

► **EXERCISE 2**

Get on all fours with legs at a 90 degree angle to the upper body (A). Draw the buttocks back to the heels and, at the same time, extend the left arm out in front, while your forehead is resting on your right arm (B). Stretch out the right arm further, and hold the position. Relax; repeat with the opposite arm.

A

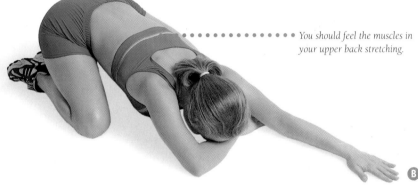

You should feel the muscles in your upper back stretching.

B

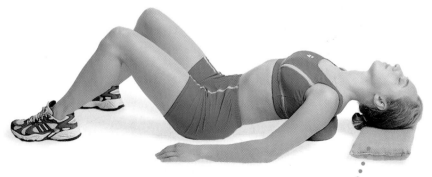

► **EXERCISE 3**

Lie on the floor with your knees bent at a 90 degree angle and your feet flat on the floor. Between your shoulder blades, place a small ball or a rolled-up towel; hold this position for 10 seconds.

The pillow supports the neck so as not to strain it.

Neck Area

▶ **EXERCISE 1**

Lie down with your knees bent and your hands clasped behind your head (A). Exhaling, bring your elbows together (as for a sit-up) and raise your head with your arms, bringing the chin close to the chest (B). Hold this position, relax, and repeat.

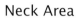

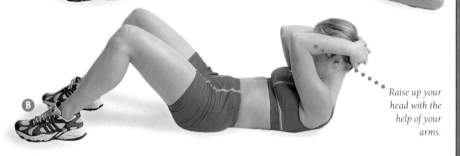

Raise up your head with the help of your arms.

▶ **EXERCISE 2**

Sit in a chair with your feet firmly on the ground, hands behind the neck, and fingers interlaced (A). Exhaling, bring the head forward, letting it fall under the weight of the arms (B). Hold the position. Return to the starting position, and repeat.

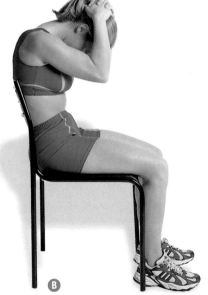

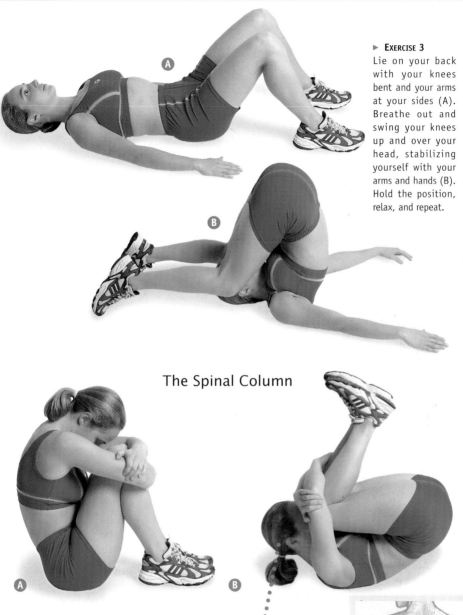

▶ **EXERCISE 3**
Lie on your back with your knees bent and your arms at your sides (A). Breathe out and swing your knees up and over your head, stabilizing yourself with your arms and hands (B). Hold the position, relax, and repeat.

The Spinal Column

Keep your head forward, nested between your knees.

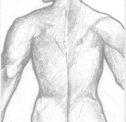

▶ **EXERCISE 1**
Sit on the floor and hug your legs close to your body, your head bent forward between your knees (A). Breathe in; exhale and start to roll backward, reaching the neck zone, and then return to a sitting position (B). Repeat.

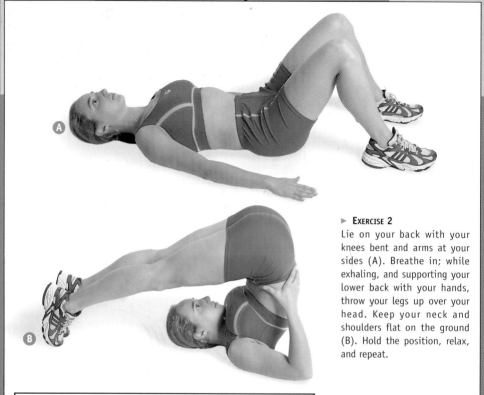

▶ **EXERCISE 2**
Lie on your back with your knees bent and arms at your sides (A). Breathe in; while exhaling, and supporting your lower back with your hands, throw your legs up over your head. Keep your neck and shoulders flat on the ground (B). Hold the position, relax, and repeat.

WORK OUT ON A FLAT SURFACE THAT ALLOWS YOU TO EXERCISE COMFORTABLY, WITHOUT PAIN AND WITHOUT HINDERING YOUR MOVEMENTS.

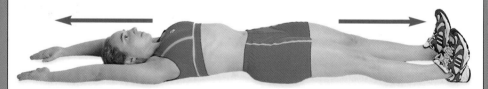

▶ **EXERCISE 3**
Stretch yourself out on the floor on your back, legs spread slightly apart and arms reaching over your head, palms upward. Extend your legs, and keep your toes pointed up. Breathe in; then exhale, actively pushing your heels down and stretching your arms over your head. Relax and repeat. While stretching, try not to curve your lower back.

Do not arch your lower back!

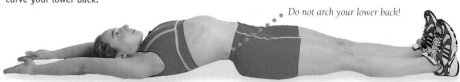

Abdominal Muscle Network
Central Abdominals

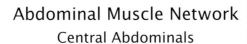

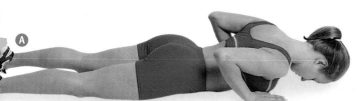

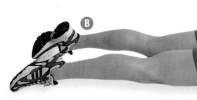

▶ EXERCISE 1

Lie flat on your stomach with your arms bent and your hands supporting your weight, under your shoulders (A). Breathing out, lift up with your arms, raising your chest off the floor without moving your pelvis (B). Hold the position, relax, and repeat.

▶ EXERCISE 2

Starting from the same position as for Exercise 1, this time hyperextend your head, looking up at the ceiling, in order to further stretch the abdominal muscles. Hold the position, relax, and repeat.

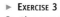

▶ EXERCISE 3

In the same position as for the preceding exercise, hyperextend the neck area, but this time raise your legs up toward your head, bending them behind you. Hold the position, relax, and repeat.

65

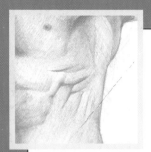

Side (Oblique) Abdominals

▶ **EXERCISE 1**

Stand with your legs spread slightly apart and your arms raised over your head (A). Bend your upper body toward the left by reaching your right arm over your head and moving your left arm down at your side. Exhaling, slide your left arm down, toward your left foot, and stretch your right arm further to the side (B). Hold this position, relax, and repeat with the other side.

▶ **EXERCISE 2**

Lie supine on the floor with your neck supported by a cushion, arms slightly apart (A). Bend your left leg and swing it over your right, grasping your left knee with your right hand. At the same time, twist your head and torso toward the left (B). While breathing out, hold the position, maintaining light pressure with your hand. Relax; repeat on the other side.

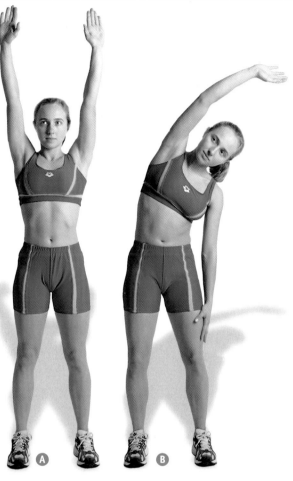

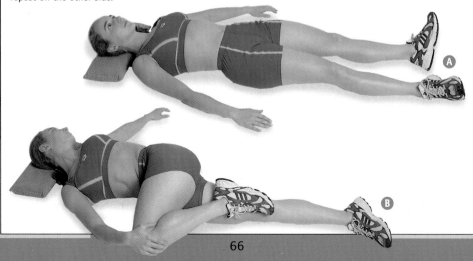

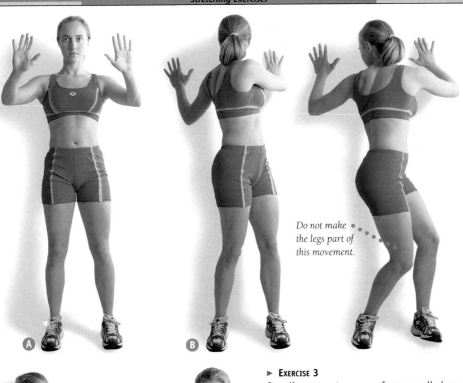

Do not make the legs part of this movement.

▶ **EXERCISE 3**

Standing one step away from a wall, legs slightly apart, raise your hands in front of you with your elbows bent (A). Exhaling, twist your upper body around, trying to touch the wall behind you with your hands (B). Hold the position, relax, and repeat in the opposite direction. During this exercise, while twisting your upper body, neither the pelvis nor the legs should move.

Pectorals

▶ **EXERCISE 1**

Stand with your right side touching the wall and right arm extended behind you, also in contact with the wall (A). While exhaling, turn your body toward the left, trying to look toward your hand on the wall (B). Hold the position, relax, and repeat on the opposite side.

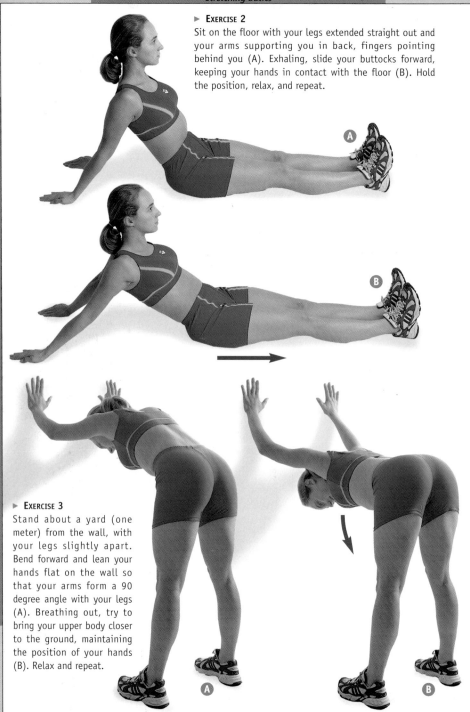

▶ **EXERCISE 2**

Sit on the floor with your legs extended straight out and your arms supporting you in back, fingers pointing behind you (A). Exhaling, slide your buttocks forward, keeping your hands in contact with the floor (B). Hold the position, relax, and repeat.

▶ **EXERCISE 3**

Stand about a yard (one meter) from the wall, with your legs slightly apart. Bend forward and lean your hands flat on the wall so that your arms form a 90 degree angle with your legs (A). Breathing out, try to bring your upper body closer to the ground, maintaining the position of your hands (B). Relax and repeat.

Deltoids

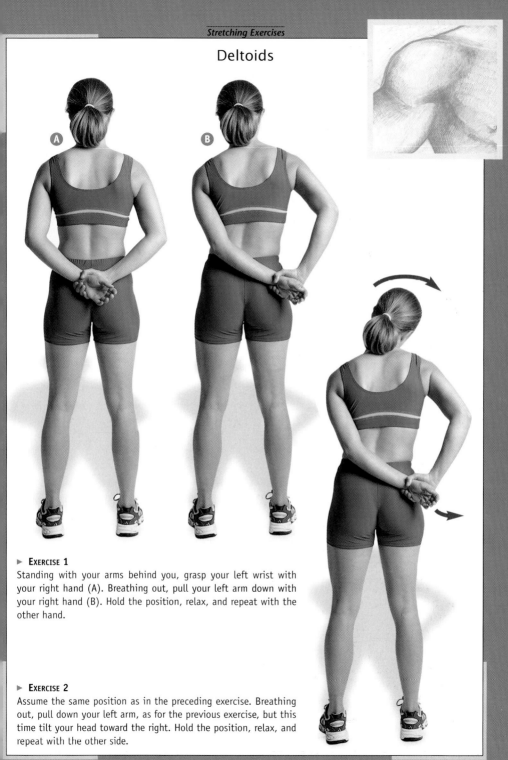

▶ **EXERCISE 1**

Standing with your arms behind you, grasp your left wrist with your right hand (A). Breathing out, pull your left arm down with your right hand (B). Hold the position, relax, and repeat with the other hand.

▶ **EXERCISE 2**

Assume the same position as in the preceding exercise. Breathing out, pull down your left arm, as for the previous exercise, but this time tilt your head toward the right. Hold the position, relax, and repeat with the other side.

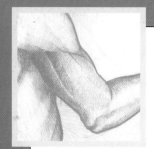

Triceps

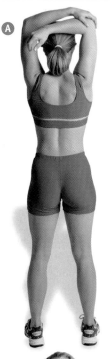

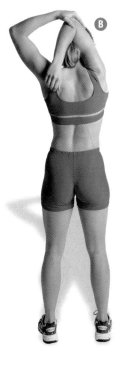

▶ **EXERCISE 1**
Stand with your arms folded over your head, draping your left hand over your right elbow (A). Exhaling, bend your right arm down behind your back (B). Hold the position; repeat with the other arm.

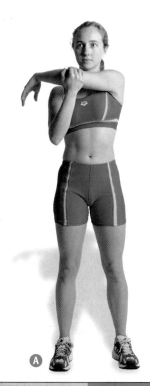

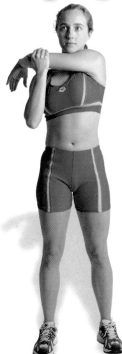

▶ **EXERCISE 2**
Stand with your left arm raised and bent, elbow pointing in front of you, supported by your right hand (A). Exhale, pulling your left arm toward your chest, applying slow and steady pressure inward with your right arm (B). Hold the position, relax, and repeat with the other side.

Shoulders

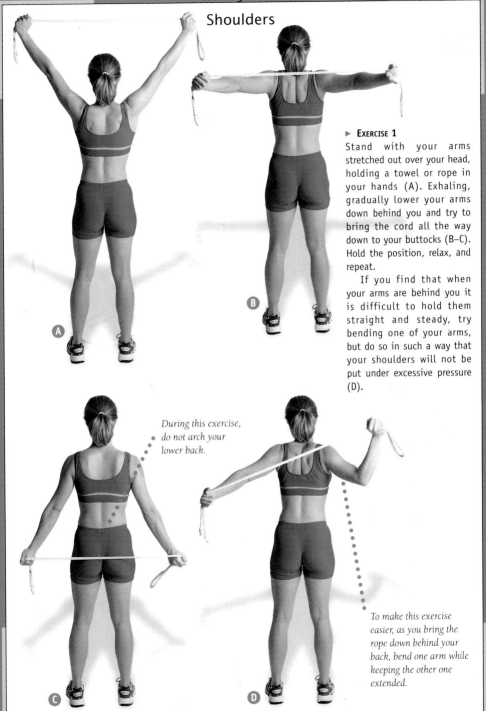

▶ **EXERCISE 1**
Stand with your arms stretched out over your head, holding a towel or rope in your hands (A). Exhaling, gradually lower your arms down behind you and try to bring the cord all the way down to your buttocks (B–C). Hold the position, relax, and repeat.

If you find that when your arms are behind you it is difficult to hold them straight and steady, try bending one of your arms, but do so in such a way that your shoulders will not be put under excessive pressure (D).

During this exercise, do not arch your lower back.

To make this exercise easier, as you bring the rope down behind your back, bend one arm while keeping the other one extended.

▶ EXERCISE 2

Stand with your right arm bent behind you, elbow pointed up, and your left arm bent behind you, elbow pointing down (A). While exhaling, try to join your hands behind your back by reaching down with your right arm and up with your left (B). Hold the position, relax, and repeat on the other side.

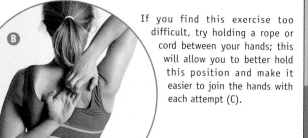

If you find this exercise too difficult, try holding a rope or cord between your hands; this will allow you to better hold this position and make it easier to join the hands with each attempt (C).

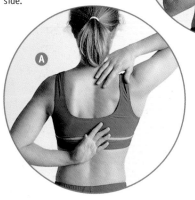

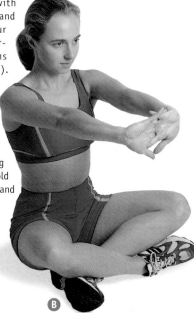

Arms

▶ EXERCISE 1

Sit on the floor with your legs crossed and your hands in your lap, fingers interlaced and palms facing inward (A). Exhaling, extend your arms up and forward, turning your hands so that your palms face outward, but without loosening your fingers (B). Hold this position, relax, and repeat.

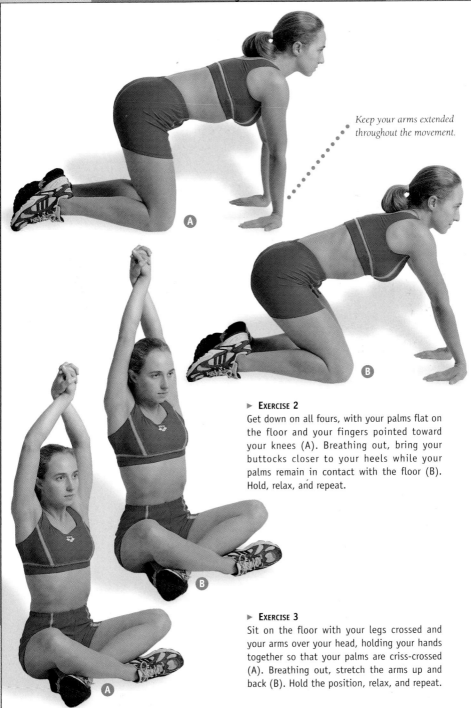

Keep your arms extended throughout the movement.

▶ **EXERCISE 2**
Get down on all fours, with your palms flat on the floor and your fingers pointed toward your knees (A). Breathing out, bring your buttocks closer to your heels while your palms remain in contact with the floor (B). Hold, relax, and repeat.

▶ **EXERCISE 3**
Sit on the floor with your legs crossed and your arms over your head, holding your hands together so that your palms are criss-crossed (A). Breathing out, stretch the arms up and back (B). Hold the position, relax, and repeat.

Fingers and Wrists

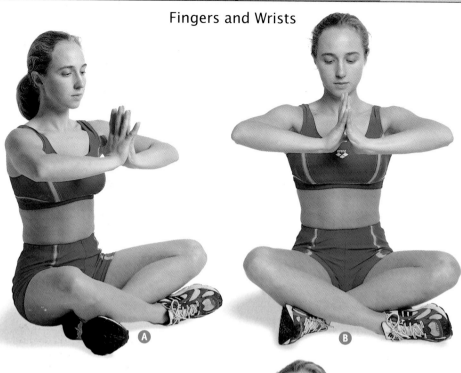

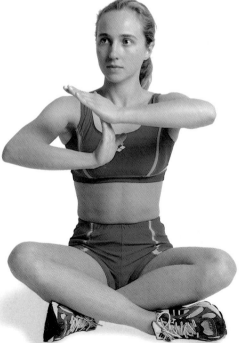

▶ **EXERCISE 1**
Sit on the floor with your legs crossed and elbows bent outward, with your palms meeting at chest level (A). Breathe out, keeping your fingertips together while spreading the palms apart. During this movement, press your fingers together in order to stretch them (B). Hold this position, relax, and repeat.

▶ **EXERCISE 2**
Sit on the floor with your legs crossed. Raising your arms to chest level, elbows bent to the sides, touch the palm of your left hand with the fingers of your right hand. While breathing out, push the fingers of your right hand toward the left forearm. Hold this position, relax, and repeat with the opposite hand.

The Face

The use of stretching for the purpose of facial care could prove to be truly important—above all, because it is the face that shows evidence of the tension and stress that characterize our daily lives. Exercising the muscles of the mouth, cheeks, neck, forehead, and eye sockets helps your face to stay relaxed and toned: even the most expensive and renowned beauty cream could never give you the same results.

▶ **EXERCISE 1**
Sitting with your arms relaxed at your sides, breathe out while opening your mouth as wide as possible and sticking your tongue out, over your chin. Relax and repeat (A).

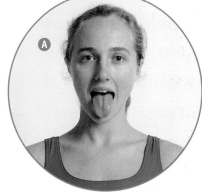

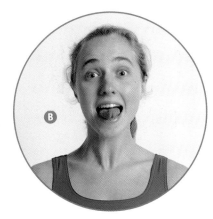

▶ **EXERCISE 2**
Sit with your arms relaxed at your sides. Breathing out, try to open your mouth, sticking your tongue straight out, and at the same time opening your eyes as wide as possible. For this exercise it is helpful to let out an "Aaah" sound. Hold, relax, and repeat (B).

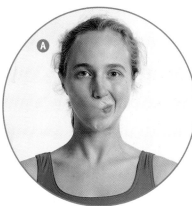

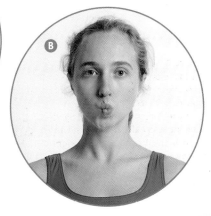

▶ **EXERCISE 3**
Sitting with your arms relaxed at your sides, purse your lips and move your mouth to the right, to the left (A), and then forward (B), alternating among the three different positions.

75

Stretching and...

STRETCHING AND ATHLETIC TRAINING

Stretching is now a regular part of the workout programs that sports trainers manage, although one may remark here that, even if the intention is a good one, the process is not always well thought-out. For athletes operating at a high performance level, stretching plays an important role in preparation and in staying in shape, both during and after an activity (whether professional or amateur). There are three main reasons for this:

▶ The first is that stretching leads to muscle flexibility, and consequently, to greater freedom of movement. This requirement is vital for all sports activities, and in particular, for certain of them like martial arts and dance, where stretching is of fundamental importance.

▶ The second, which as yet has no precise classification, involves the role of stretching before games and competitions. Let us remember that, on the physiological level, stretching stimulates circulation in the capillaries of the muscles, producing a "pump effect" that sends blood to the muscle veins and fibers. This obviates strain and possible harm to the tissues.

Lengthening itself during exercise, the muscle stretches and compresses, thereby clearing out the blood and lymph system; this can be compared to a sponge that, when pressed, rids itself of water. When an exercise is completed, the muscle relaxes—the negative pressure that ensues then facilitates blood flow back into the muscle.

Such processes give rise to a feeling of warmth and energy that prepares the muscle for the exertion required by athletic activity—above all, when that very muscle, in situations largely dependent on the athletes' emotional state, runs the risk of losing some of its tone.

▶ The third matter is the winding down period. This aspect is often forgotten either by the athletes or their trainers. Preoccupied by the warm-up and stretching before the game and by the outcome, one forgets to remind the athlete or physical education student to stretch one last time at the end of the activity. Stretching practiced after the execution of the prescribed exercises or game corrects the imbalance that such muscular activity tends to create, and helps eliminate excess substances produced from muscle work during exertion (notably lactic acid and other metabolites).

By stimulating the circulation, the lactic acid that has built up can be removed. This biological by-product is produced especially

Applying stretching during athletic training improves performance and helps prevent injurious accidents.

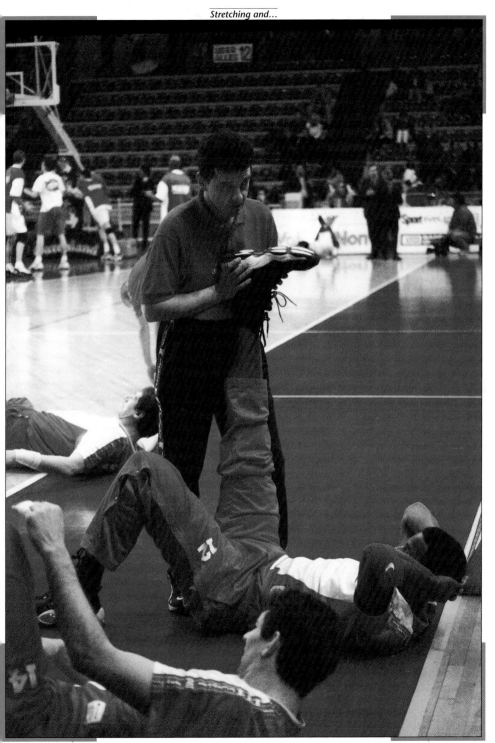

	Exercises	Number
TENNIS	Ankles	3
	Calves	2, 3
	Thighs	2
	Quadriceps	1, 2, 3, 5
	Thigh and hip	1, 4
	Lower back	1, 2
	Upper back	1, 2
	Neck area	1
	Triceps	1, 2
	Pectorals	1, 2
	Arms	1, 2
	Fingers and wrists	2
	Shoulders	1, 2

	Exercises	Number
BASKETBALL AND VOLLEYBALL	Ankles	2
	Calves	2, 4
	Thighs	3, 4
	Quadriceps	2, 3, 4, 5
	Thigh and hip	2, 3
	Lower back	2, 3
	Upper back	2, 3
	Neck area	1
	Triceps	1
	Pectorals	1
	Arms	1, 2, 3
	Fingers and wrists	1, 2
	Shoulders	1, 2

	Exercises	Number
SOCCER	Ankles	1, 3
	Calves	1, 4
	Thighs	1, 4
	Quadriceps	1, 2, 4, 5
	Thigh and hip	1, 4
	Lower back	1
	Spinal column	1, 3
	Abdominal muscles	1, 2
	Arms	1, 3
	Shoulders	1, 2

	Exercises	Number
TRACK	Feet	3
	Ankles	1, 3, 4
	Calves	1, 2, 4
	Thighs	1, 4
	Quadriceps	1, 2, 5
	Thigh and hip	1, 2
	Lower back	2, 4
	Spinal column	1, 3
	Triceps	1
	Pectorals	1

when performing deep-breathing exercises, such as aerobics. Whether or not you are an athlete, getting in the habit of carrying out stretching exercises after muscular exertion will yield positive effects—especially in the days immediately following.

In this way, the muscles will not give in so easily to the sore feeling that is the norm after an exercise or activity that may not have been practiced for a while.

Including a good winding-down routine with your stretching will accustom you to training and sports activities more quickly, with better results, and with fewer possibilities of developing muscle traumas.

STRETCHING AND PAIN

Rigidity is something all of us engaged in exercise regimens are familiar with. It can arise

SWIMMING	Exercises	Number
	Ankles	2
	Calves	2, 4
	Thighs	3, 4
	Quadriceps	2, 3, 4, 5
	Thigh and hip	2, 3
	Lower back	2, 3
	Upper back	2, 3
	Neck area	1
	Abdominal muscles	1, 4
	Triceps	1
	Pectorals	1
	Arms	1, 2, 3
	Shoulders	1, 2

WEIGHT LIFTING	Exercises	Number
	Calves	1, 2
	Thighs	1, 2
	Quadriceps	1, 2
	Thigh and hip	1
	Lower back	1, 3
	Upper back	1, 2
	Neck area	1
	Abdominal muscles	1, 3
	Deltoids	1
	Triceps	1, 2
	Arms	1, 3
	Shoulders	1, 2

CYCLING	Exercises	Number
	Ankles	2
	Calves	2, 4
	Thighs	3, 4
	Quadriceps	2, 3, 4
	Hips	2, 3
	Lower back	2, 3
	Upper back	2, 3
	Neck area	1
	Spinal column	3
	Triceps	1

The Winding-Down Program

The tables seen on these pages indicate the sequence of stretching exercises for concluding a physical workout, based on what sport is being practiced.

• •

from stress, either emotional or physical. Think, for example, of how we feel when we are afraid. Under various circumstances, and especially under pressure, the body tends to stiffen in an unnatural way in order to inhibit or relieve painful sensations: one stiffens in order to defend oneself from a blow or to lessen, or avoid, an imminently painful situation.

The body thus creates for itself a kind of armor that is able to defend one and even repair itself in autonomous fashion, but that unfortunately makes one live in a constant state of tension that results in pain.

The parts that are most affected by such rigidity vary from person to person. There are those who are more sensitive in the spinal column and therefore experience rigidity in the neck, abdomen, and back; there are those who are quite vulnerable in the shoulders, wrists, and hands; and finally, some experience tension in the knee joints and ankles. It should also be understood that rigidity can permeate the entire body.

Such conditions can lead to inflammation in other parts of the body, which in time can degenerate and cause grave pathologies, such as arthritis. One is often not aware of such conditions until movements become limited or the symptoms of pain become too acute. For example, in the morning you may find it difficult to get up owing to a feeling of heaviness, as though you have not rested at all during the night. Or perhaps some simple physical activity like carrying home a bag of groceries causes undue fatigue, or even pain; if so, one should look into the matter.

Stiffness is often taken for granted because it is believed that it invariably appears during middle age. Many people adopt a passive attitude toward it and feel that it is useless to combat it; for this reason, it is important to work on oneself at an earlier stage in life, for by doing so, it is much easier to prevent the symptoms that come with aging. Taking no steps to avert such stiffening is a wrong approach, because a well thought-out exercise routine can help prevent any number of complaints as well as keep one in optimal shape.

Below are some tables of exercises germane

> Although stretching on a regular basis is important, doing it well is even more crucial. Such exercise relaxes the muscles and helps rid them of accumulated tension.

	Exercises	Number
TROUBLE SPOTS	Feet	1, 2
	Ankles	1, 2, 3
	Knees	3
	Hips	1, 3
	Lower back	1, 2, 3
	Upper back	1, 3
	Neck area	1, 2, 3
	Shoulders	1 (with towel), 2
	Hands	1, 2

The table above contains some suggestions for specific exercises. These should be carried out with care, making it a point not to apply more force than necessary. The exercises are geared to the specific areas of the body that are liable to be affected by rigidity.

> Stress and nervous tension tend to stiffen the body, making certain stretching techniques more difficult to apply. Before you start, try to relax.

Insomnia

One of the principal objectives of stretching is to help the body relax and, over time, maintain a calm physiological state. There are several suggested exercises that will help achieve such a goal and prevent anxious states of mind, such as those that lead to insomnia. As we pointed out in the chapter dealing with the role of respiration, the exhalation phase of breathing makes muscle and mental release possible, thereby inducing a state of self-relaxation.

Consequently, the given exercises will be more useful if carried out while stretched out on the ground, though they might seem easier to perform in bed. While referring to the information dealing with respiration (see page 24, it is advisable to carry out the following:

	Exercises	Number
INSOMNIA	Gluteals	1, 2, 3
	Side (oblique) abdominals	2

> Working on some stretching exercises before retiring for the night will lead to better and sounder sleep.

SPECIFIC STRETCHING: ZEROING IN ON THE NEUROMUSCULAR CENTERS

The Proprioceptive Neuromuscular Facilitation (PNF) method was developed in the 1940s and drawn up in 1950, in the United States. It deals primarily with neuromotor activity and function.

This method cannot be considered a stretching technique in the strict sense, as

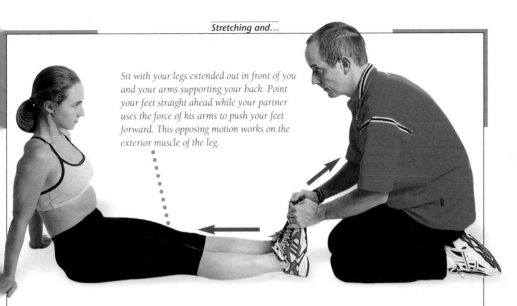

Sit with your legs extended out in front of you and your arms supporting your back. Point your feet straight ahead while your partner uses the force of his arms to push your feet forward. This opposing motion works on the exterior muscle of the leg.

much as a combination of isometric contractions and muscular relaxations. This system is based on the conclusions of many research studies dealing with what happens immediately after an isometric contraction (a contraction in which a muscle exerts force but does not change in length). Following such a contraction, these studies found, one has a spontaneous decrease in muscle tone, thereby permitting passive stretching techniques to work more efficiently.

In order to follow up on the previous suggestions with regard to passive stretching, one will need the assistance of a partner who, if not an expert, at least has some basic knowledge of working out the muscles. We will now present a course of exercise involving two people. These may help clarify, albeit briefly, the concepts introduced above.

On the following pages we will present series of detailed exercises that will give you illustrated instructions to carry out exercises in specific situations and circumstances.

The cooperation of two people creates the conditions necessary for carrying out muscle contractions geared toward specific regions of the body.

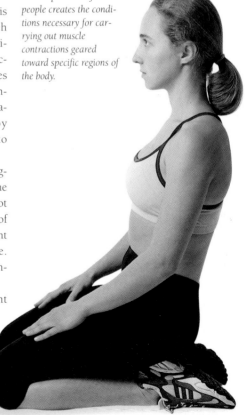

Stretching in Pairs

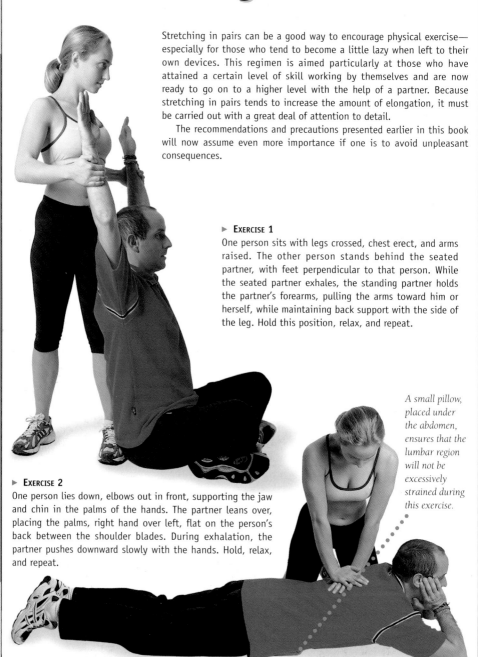

Stretching in pairs can be a good way to encourage physical exercise—especially for those who tend to become a little lazy when left to their own devices. This regimen is aimed particularly at those who have attained a certain level of skill working by themselves and are now ready to go on to a higher level with the help of a partner. Because stretching in pairs tends to increase the amount of elongation, it must be carried out with a great deal of attention to detail.

The recommendations and precautions presented earlier in this book will now assume even more importance if one is to avoid unpleasant consequences.

► **EXERCISE 1**

One person sits with legs crossed, chest erect, and arms raised. The other person stands behind the seated partner, with feet perpendicular to that person. While the seated partner exhales, the standing partner holds the partner's forearms, pulling the arms toward him or herself, while maintaining back support with the side of the leg. Hold this position, relax, and repeat.

A small pillow, placed under the abdomen, ensures that the lumbar region will not be excessively strained during this exercise.

► **EXERCISE 2**

One person lies down, elbows out in front, supporting the jaw and chin in the palms of the hands. The partner leans over, placing the palms, right hand over left, flat on the person's back between the shoulder blades. During exhalation, the partner pushes downward slowly with the hands. Hold, relax, and repeat.

► **EXERCISE 3**

One person lies down on her back with the left leg bent and the right leg extended up. The partner holds her foot, pressing it into his abdomen (A). The person standing pushes the extended leg for-ward very slowly, like a lever, while the partner, during exhalation, resists his pressure (B). Hold the position, relax, and repeat with the other leg.

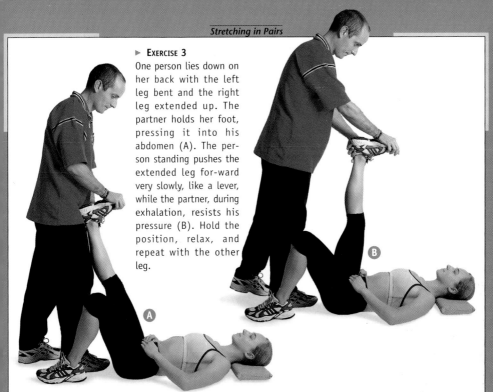

► **EXERCISE 4**

One person stands in back of the other. The person in front bends his legs, grasps the wrists of the person behind, leaning over and lifting her onto his back like a sack of flour (A). The person in back lies on her stomach on the partner's back in a relaxed position (B). While returning her to the ground, the legs should be positioned in such a way that the weight is distributed evenly, and does not cause back pain or strain.

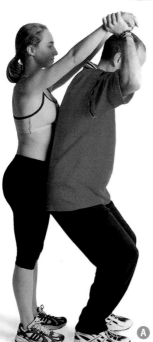

Stretching and Pregnancy

During pregnancy, a woman's body undergoes so many changes, that to make a list of them would require us to write a specialized book. Keep in mind, however, that certain hormones (e.g., progesterone and relaxin) work to relax and soften the ligaments and to permit greater mobility—above all, of the pelvis—which makes childbirth easier. This physiological change puts a woman in a position to apply stretching techniques from which she will quickly derive valuable benefits.

As already explained, you should choose a time that is the most conducive to start stretching, wear comfortable clothing, and concentrate fully on your body. It is also important, from the beginning, to pay fuller attention to breathing and its correct application during the exercise. "Let yourself go" in order to get in touch with your innermost sensations; do not become discouraged if you feel that you are simply "too heavy." Instead, take advantage of the new condition in which you find yourself, for it allows you to attain and maintain results that you would otherwise have to work harder for.

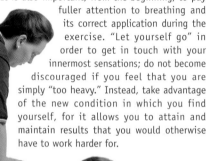

You must not thrust your back up in the air or bring your head down suddenly; instead, work in a smooth and gentle fashion.

▶ **EXERCISE 1**
Get down on all fours (A). Exhale deeply, allowing your chest to sag down, and raise your head (B). Then inhale, gently arching your back upward and lowering your head (C). Hold each position in turn, relax, and repeat.

► **EXERCISE 2**

Starting from a standing position with your legs spread slightly apart (A), try while exhaling to bring your buttocks closer to the floor, keeping your heels to the floor (B). Hold this position, return to the standing position, and repeat. This exercise can be simplified by placing a pile of books or a thick cushion on the floor (C).

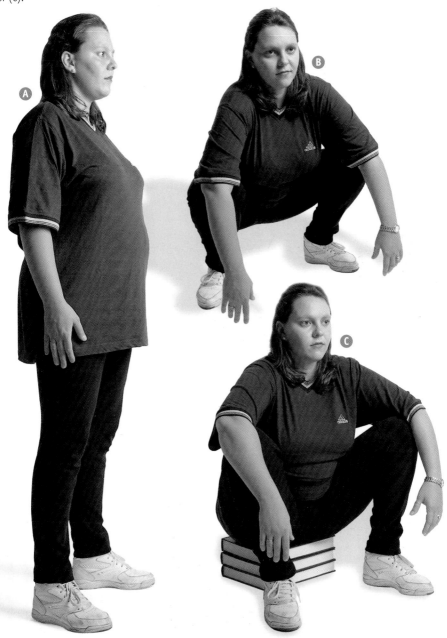

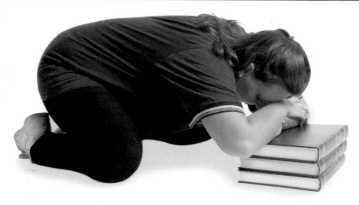

▶ EXERCISE 3

Place your hands on top of a stack of books. Crouch so that your head is resting on top of your hands, while folding your legs and arms under you. Your knees should be spread apart and your chest should be toward the floor. Hold this position, relax, and repeat.

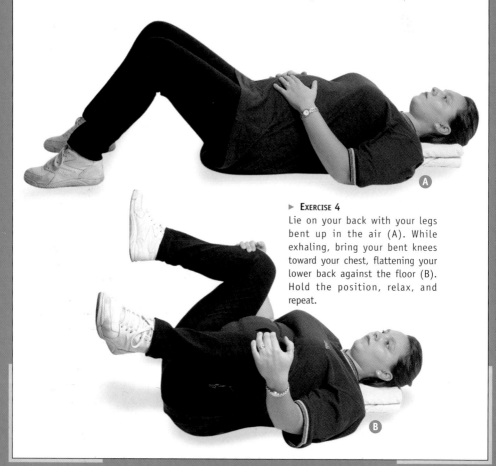

▶ EXERCISE 4

Lie on your back with your legs bent up in the air (A). While exhaling, bring your bent knees toward your chest, flattening your lower back against the floor (B). Hold the position, relax, and repeat.

► **EXERCISE 5**

Slowly and carefully, from a supine position, bring your legs up against a wall. Once you are able to hold this position (perhaps by placing a pillow under the buttocks), carry out the following movements.

Position a pillow under the buttocks to help you maintain this posture.

A. While exhaling, reach back with your arms on the floor; stretch your heels up against the wall. Hold the position, relax, and repeat.

B. Keeping your arms extended behind you, exhale and spread your legs apart while keeping your heels against the wall. Hold, relax, and repeat.

C. Bring the soles of your feet together by bending your legs towards your pelvis, and place your hands on the inside of your thighs. Exhale, pressing down lightly on your thighs. Hold, relax, and repeat.

Stretching for Seniors

If you think that stretching is appropriate only for the young and the athletic, and not for those of mature years, then you are mistaken. This misconception prevents many older people from taking full advantage of the benefits of stretching.

Stretching gives seniors the sense of controlling their exercise activity—experiencing the intensity of the exercise, but above all, directing the movements of the body as a whole. This allows the elderly to take on this work with a positive attitude, and almost guarantees renewed well-being in the following ways:
—Maintaining healthy joint mobility;
—Improving posture, as well as helping to prevent the onset of bad posture that is typical at older ages;
—Maintaining elasticity and mobility of the torso (including the ribcage and breathing apparatus), with consequent improvement in respiratory function; and
—Imparting a feeling of increased mental and physical well-being.

All of these improvements also affect the psychological health of an elderly person, who often tends to feel abandoned and alone. Instead, an elderly person engaged in stretching tends to "stay in shape" in all senses of the phrase.

▶ EXERCISE 1
Get down on all fours (A), exhale, and bring your buttocks back on your heels (B). Hold the position, relax, and repeat.

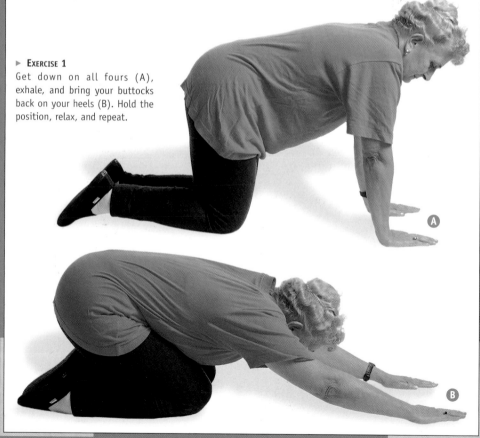

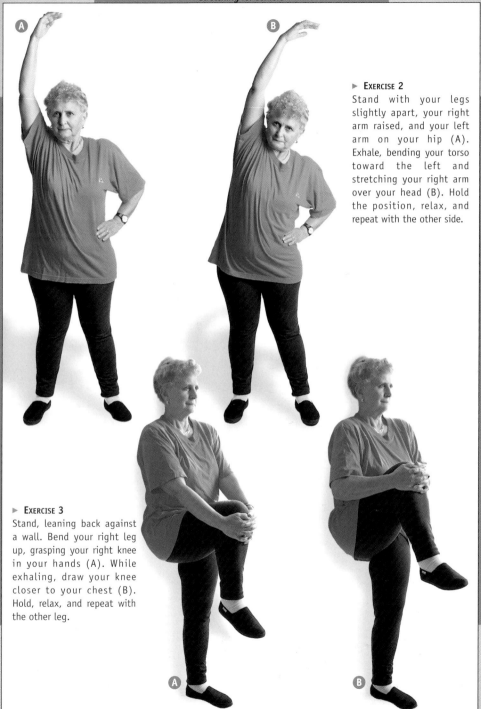

▶ **EXERCISE 2**
Stand with your legs slightly apart, your right arm raised, and your left arm on your hip (A). Exhale, bending your torso toward the left and stretching your right arm over your head (B). Hold the position, relax, and repeat with the other side.

▶ **EXERCISE 3**
Stand, leaning back against a wall. Bend your right leg up, grasping your right knee in your hands (A). While exhaling, draw your knee closer to your chest (B). Hold, relax, and repeat with the other leg.

▶ **EXERCISE 4**

While seated on the floor, lean up against a wall, extending your right leg in front of you and grasping your right foot with your hands (A). Breathing out, bring your right leg up, closer to your chest (B). Hold this position, relax, and repeat with other leg.

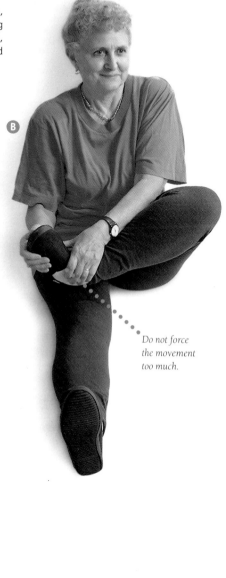

B

Do not force the movement too much.

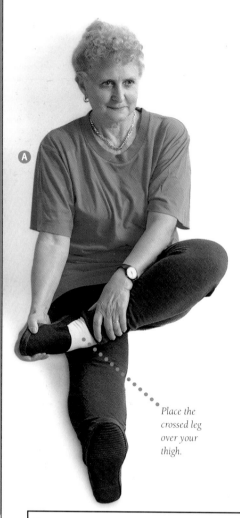

A

Place the crossed leg over your thigh.

PERFORMING STRETCHING EXERCISES DURING THE ADVANCED YEARS WILL SLOW DOWN THE EFFECTS OF AGING, WHICH INEVITABLY AFFECT THE MUSCLES AND JOINTS.

Stretching for Musicians

It may seem rather strange to talk about stretching exercises to help musicians, but when combining these two disciplines, it is not hard to understand how they go together. There are in fact two ways in which music is linked to athletic activity.

The first has to do with the employment of positions that are not always correct, and that oblige the musician to hold a posture for a long time—with a great risk of bodily harm. The neck area for violinists and flute players, the elbows for harp players, and the lower back (which may become unnecessarily curved) for piano players are only a few examples of places where harm may result from maintaining incorrect positions over long periods of time.

The second aspect (closely related to the previous one) refers to the hours of practice time that every musician must invest to improve his or her technique. This rigorous discipline may lead to nonphysical conditions that begin to affect the body in unknown ways. Just as in the sporting world, in the music field one finds oneself in a specialization that makes demands on the entire body. Therefore, one can easily see how stretching exercises should become a part of every musician's daily work routine. Furthermore, it is notable that in conservatories, only a few teachers apprise their students of how to sit properly so as to avoid the discomfort of holding a posture for too long. In the following pages, we present exercises specifically tailored to the players of selected musical instruments.

Violin

For the violinist that accumulates tension in the top part of the chest, we suggest some exercises that are adapted mainly to the neck area and to the upper body. In addition, exercises for the hands and fingers should be undertaken (see page 37).

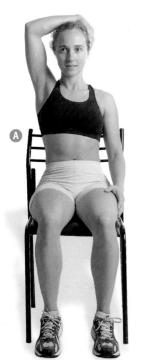

Ⓐ

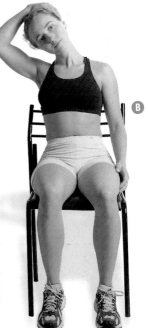

Ⓑ

▶ **EXERCISE 1**
While seated, place your right hand on top of your head with your fingers touching your left ear (A). Breathing out, tilt your head to the right, helping with your right hand (B). Hold this position, relax, and repeat with the other side.

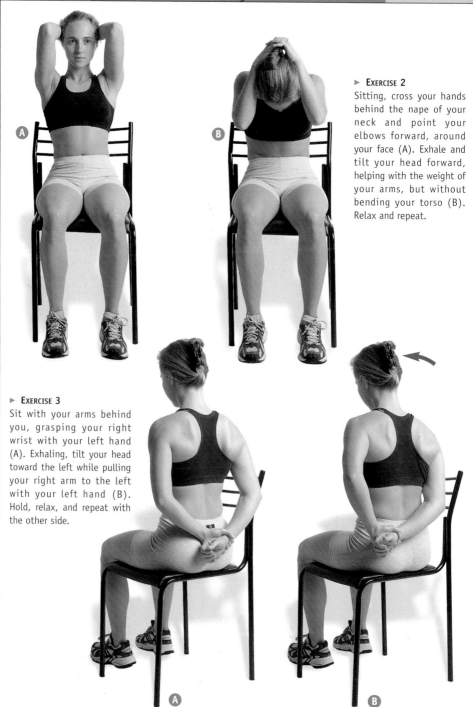

► **EXERCISE 2**
Sitting, cross your hands behind the nape of your neck and point your elbows forward, around your face (A). Exhale and tilt your head forward, helping with the weight of your arms, but without bending your torso (B). Relax and repeat.

► **EXERCISE 3**
Sit with your arms behind you, grasping your right wrist with your left hand (A). Exhaling, tilt your head toward the left while pulling your right arm to the left with your left hand (B). Hold, relax, and repeat with the other side.

Guitar

The position for playing the guitar is indeed hard on the upper body, the chest, and the arm muscles. For this reason, we recommend several exercises to limber up this muscle group.

► **EXERCISE 1**
Same as Exercise 2 for the violin.

► **EXERCISE 2**
Sit with your chest erect (A). While exhaling, bend forward, hanging your arms down over the tops of your feet (B). Try to touch your toes. Hold this position, return to the starting point, and repeat.

► **EXERCISE 3**
Sit with your arms resting on your thighs and your fingers interlaced (A). Extend your arms in front of you at chest level. While exhaling, rotate your hands so that your palms face forward (B). Release hands and repeat.

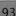

Piano

If not correctly seated while playing the piano, undue injury may occur in your neck and lower back area. All of the chest muscles, therefore, must exert themselves in order for the musculature to properly alternate between moments of work and moments of relaxation. We will also concentrate on the muscles of the fingers, which are used so intensively with this instrument.

▶ **EXERCISE 1**
Sit with your fingers interlaced and your arms resting on your thighs (A). While inhaling, extend your arms over your head, rotating your hands so that your palms face upward (B). Hold this position, return to the starting point, and repeat.

A

B

▶ **EXERCISE 2**
While seated, place your right hand on your hip. Reach your left arm over your head, slightly curved to your right side (A). While exhaling, bend your torso to the right, stretching your left arm over your head (B). Hold, relax, and repeat with the other side.

A

B

94

▶ **EXERCISE 3**
Hold your palms together, placed in front of your chest (A). While exhaling, separate your palms while pressing your fingertips together, spreading your fingers apart (B). Hold, relax, and repeat.

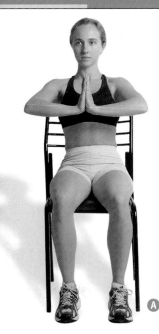

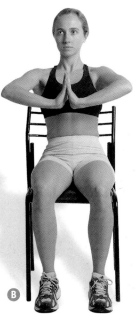

(A)

(B)

Flute

Although the flute requires a more dynamic position than the instruments already discussed, the rotation of the chest region and the work of suspending the arms call for a specialized type of stretching exercise.

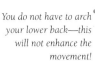

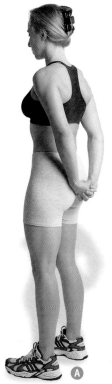

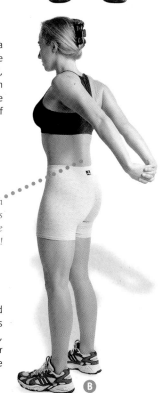

You do not have to arch your lower back—this will not enhance the movement!

▶ **EXERCISE 1**
Stand with your hands behind your back and your fingers interlaced (A). While exhaling, bring your arms up, keeping your palms facing inward (B). Hold the position, relax, and repeat.

(A)

(B)

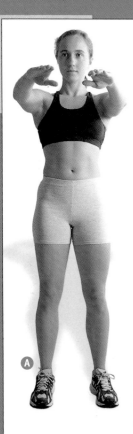

A

▶ **EXERCISE 2**
Stand with your back one yard from the wall (about a meter away). Raise your arms in front of you, keeping your upper body erect (A). While keeping the pelvis area steady, exhale, twisting your upper body to the left, until you can touch the wall with your hands (B). Hold the position, relax, and repeat with the other side.

▶ **EXERCISE 3**
Same as Exercise 2 for the violin.

B

Percussion Instruments

Playing percussion instruments, whether the tambourine or the drums, requires you to use your upper arms and your chest. For this reason, the proposed exercises focus on the upper body muscles and the arms.

A

B

▶ **EXERCISE 1**
Stand perpendicular to the wall, with your right arm outstretched and your palm against the wall, in back of you at a right angle (A). Exhaling, rotate your body to the left, trying to see the top of the hand that is firmly against the wall (B). Hold this position, relax, and repeat with the other arm.

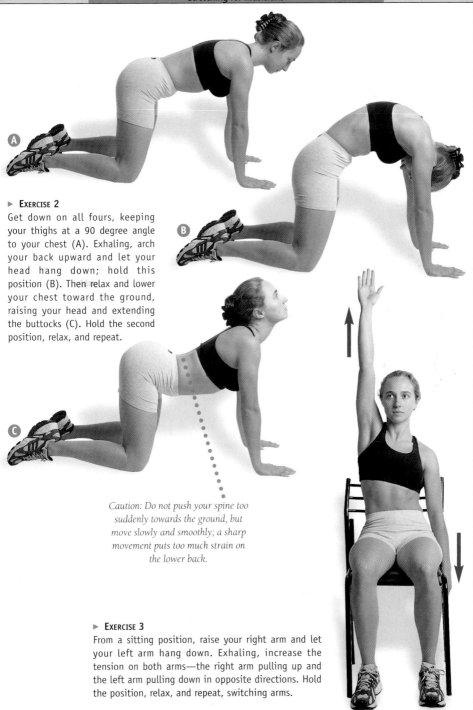

▶ **EXERCISE 2**

Get down on all fours, keeping your thighs at a 90 degree angle to your chest (A). Exhaling, arch your back upward and let your head hang down; hold this position (B). Then relax and lower your chest toward the ground, raising your head and extending the buttocks (C). Hold the second position, relax, and repeat.

Caution: Do not push your spine too suddenly towards the ground, but move slowly and smoothly; a sharp movement puts too much strain on the lower back.

▶ **EXERCISE 3**

From a sitting position, raise your right arm and let your left arm hang down. Exhaling, increase the tension on both arms—the right arm pulling up and the left arm pulling down in opposite directions. Hold the position, relax, and repeat, switching arms.

Stretching in the Office

Keeping fit while enduring the daily grind of one's job, for the majority of people, is a difficult task to accomplish. However, the performance of a few well-chosen exercises may be the solution.

Hours passed in front of a desk or a computer screen lead to a sensation of fatigue, which many people feel after a day of office work. These are the optimal conditions for developing lasting physical harm, leading to what is known as "hypokinesia" (diminished or slow movement), which gradually affects the entire body.

For this reason, performing these exercises in the middle of our day to stretch the neck, the upper back, the shoulders, the spinal column, along with the upper and lower extremities, should instill in you a sensation of well-being and a more peaceful disposition for dealing with the workday. These stretches do not require you to change clothes; rather, their application may be carried out at any time of day. These unobtrusive exercises geared to the office environment are therefore the simplest of all.

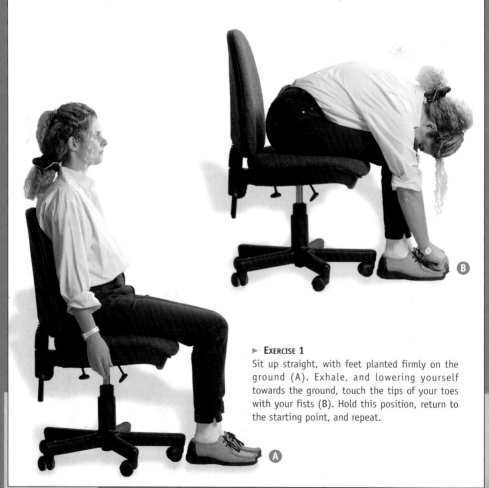

▶ **EXERCISE 1**
Sit up straight, with feet planted firmly on the ground (A). Exhale, and lowering yourself towards the ground, touch the tips of your toes with your fists (B). Hold this position, return to the starting point, and repeat.

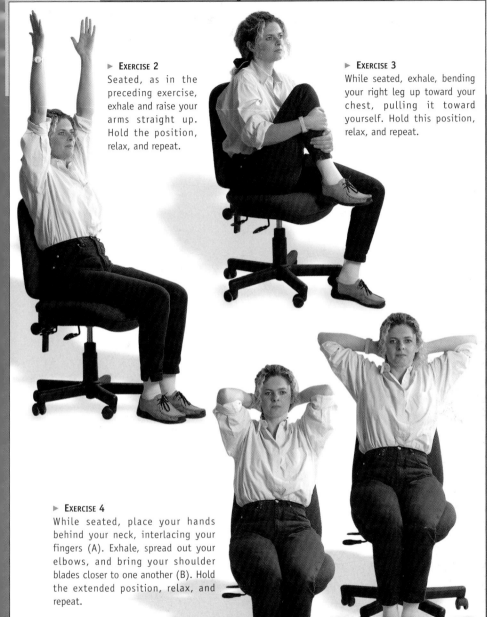

► **EXERCISE 2**
Seated, as in the preceding exercise, exhale and raise your arms straight up. Hold the position, relax, and repeat.

► **EXERCISE 3**
While seated, exhale, bending your right leg up toward your chest, pulling it toward yourself. Hold this position, relax, and repeat.

► **EXERCISE 4**
While seated, place your hands behind your neck, interlacing your fingers (A). Exhale, spread out your elbows, and bring your shoulder blades closer to one another (B). Hold the extended position, relax, and repeat.

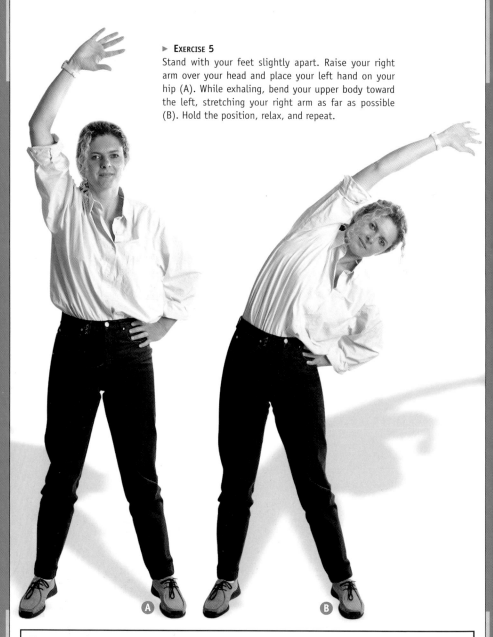

▶ **EXERCISE 5**

Stand with your feet slightly apart. Raise your right arm over your head and place your left hand on your hip (A). While exhaling, bend your upper body toward the left, stretching your right arm as far as possible (B). Hold the position, relax, and repeat.

Ⓐ   Ⓑ

THE REGULAR PRACTICE OF STRETCHING WILL ACTUALLY SAVE YOU TIME YOU WOULD HAVE LOST DUE TO FATIGUE. YOU WILL WORK MORE PRODUCTIVELY, WHILE FEELING HEALTHIER AND REJUVENATED.

Stretching
with Sports Equipment

Happily, stretching is such an inherent part (some would say the "soul") of any sport and exercise activity, that trends in clothes and equipment are hardly important considerations compared with those of getting results. Time and again, it has been affirmed that it is the stretching itself, and the results so many people obtain from it, that is the important thing. If special equipment need play any part in it, its role is strictly secondary.

To help carry out certain exercises, we can employ many informal objects that are at hand, as well as specialized gymnastics tools, such as fitness balls.

Ropes and Elastic Bands

Ropes and elastic bands have proven very useful in certain exercises (for example, where one is required to grasp the foot with one leg raised, pulling the Achilles tendons; see photo) or when one wants to increase the workload of an exercise. First of all, such equipment helps the lower back region by isolating the muscle being stretched. Secondly, correct use of such equipment can lead to better results from the proposed exercise.

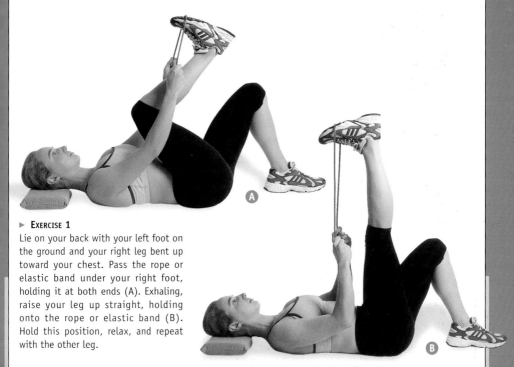

▶ **EXERCISE 1**

Lie on your back with your left foot on the ground and your right leg bent up toward your chest. Pass the rope or elastic band under your right foot, holding it at both ends (A). Exhaling, raise your leg up straight, holding onto the rope or elastic band (B). Hold this position, relax, and repeat with the other leg.

▶ **EXERCISE 2**

Sitting or standing, while still holding the elastic or rope in your hands, bring your right arm behind your head and your left arm behind your back (A). As you exhale, lightly pull up on the cord with your right hand, which raises your left hand in the process (B). Hold the position, relax, and repeat with the other arm.

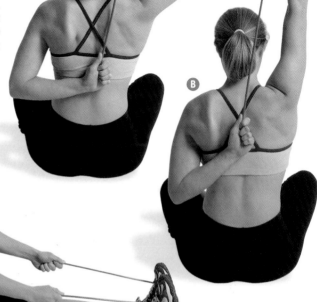

▶ **EXERCISE 3**

Sitting with your legs stretched out in front of you, hold the rope or elastic around the soles of your feet (A). Exhale; pull on the elastic with your arms, gently bringing your chest closer to your legs (B). Hold this position, relax, and repeat.

Tennis Balls

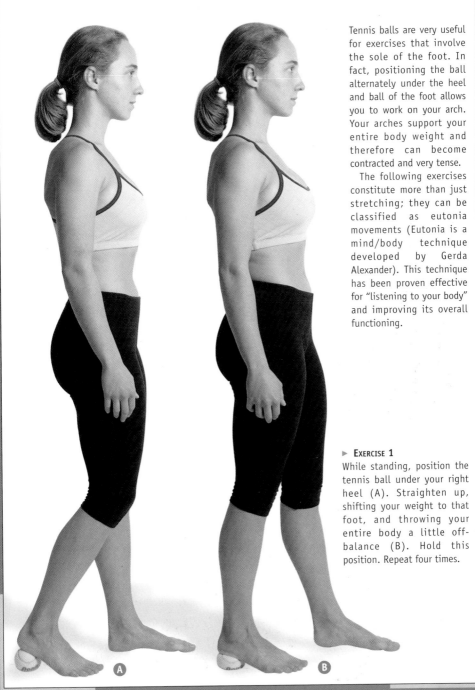

Tennis balls are very useful for exercises that involve the sole of the foot. In fact, positioning the ball alternately under the heel and ball of the foot allows you to work on your arch. Your arches support your entire body weight and therefore can become contracted and very tense.

The following exercises constitute more than just stretching; they can be classified as eutonia movements (Eutonia is a mind/body technique developed by Gerda Alexander). This technique has been proven effective for "listening to your body" and improving its overall functioning.

▶ **EXERCISE 1**
While standing, position the tennis ball under your right heel (A). Straighten up, shifting your weight to that foot, and throwing your entire body a little off-balance (B). Hold this position. Repeat four times.

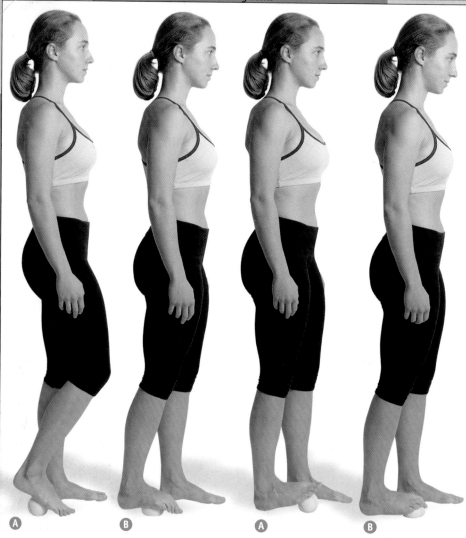

A   B   A   B

▶ **EXERCISE 2**

While standing, position the ball under the center of the arch of your right foot (A). Throwing yourself slightly off-balance, shift all of your body weight onto your right foot (B). Hold this position and repeat four times.

▶ **EXERCISE 3**

In the same position as in the preceding exercise, place the tennis ball under the ball of your foot (A). Press down firmly on it with your weight (B). Hold the position and repeat four times.

Before doing these exercises with the ball of the other foot, first place both feet on the ground so that you can feel the difference in the way the soles make contact with the floor. That done, repeat the same exercises with the left foot.

The Pull-Up Bar

The pull-up bar is applied most frequently to building upper-body muscle strength; however, it can also be utilized for stretching. While doing these hanging exercises, you will need to try to avoid incurring shoulder pains. If muscle spasms suddenly occur, you can run the risk of worsening matters. If pain persists, it is advisable to stop this form of exercise.

The bar should be placed in a doorway where you have room enough to move and turn around. Or it may be mounted on a wall where there is sufficient space to carry out the exercises.

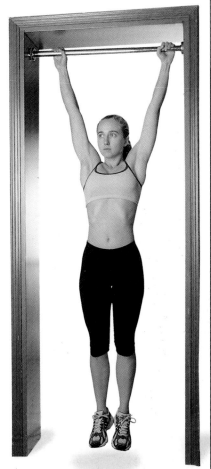

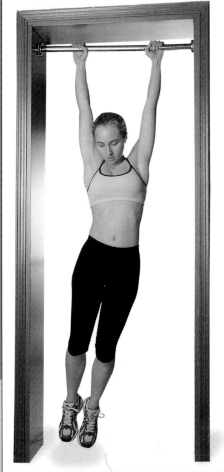

▶ **EXERCISE 1**

Hang from the bar with both hands, keeping your head relaxed between your shoulders and your legs extended. If it is too difficult to reach the bar, help yourself to climb up with a chair. While breathing in and out, try to maintain the position for 5–10 seconds. Progressively increase the duration of suspension to 30–40 seconds.

▶ **EXERCISE 2**

Hang from the bar with both hands, keeping your head relaxed between the shoulders and your legs extended. Breathing normally, swing your body to the right and then to the left. Try to keep your head and legs relaxed and free of tension. Relax and repeat, gradually increasing the time on the bar from 5–10 seconds to 30–40 seconds.

Fitness Ball

Although it is considered a plaything for children, the fitness ball is a useful and innovative tool for a variety of workouts. The exercises take advantage of the fact that thus supporting the body allows for full relaxation and extension.

The ball does not need to be inflated completely. A ball with more "give" will permit you to stabilize yourself with the help of your hands and feet.

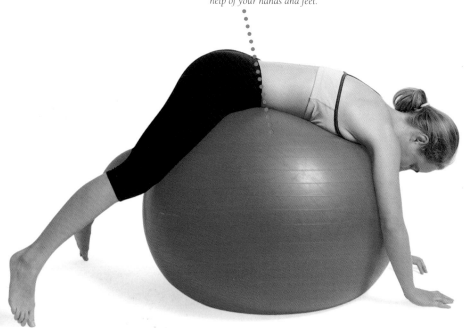

▶ **EXERCISE 1**
Drape yourself over the ball, face down, stabilizing yourself with your hands and feet. Relax your head, back, and buttocks, and breathe normally. Hold this position and repeat, increasing the duration of relaxation (from 10 seconds to 60 seconds).

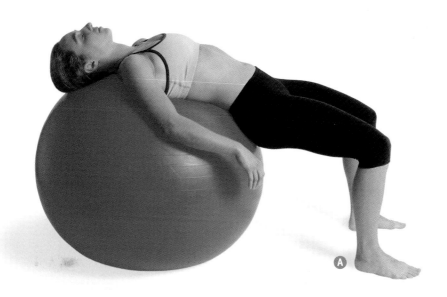

▶ **EXERCISE 2**

Lean back on the ball with your head and upper back draped over the top. Keep your feet flat on the floor with your legs bent at a 90-degree angle and your arms hanging loosely at your sides (A). Inhale; then exhale, bringing your arms up and back over your head (B). Hold this position, relax, and repeat.

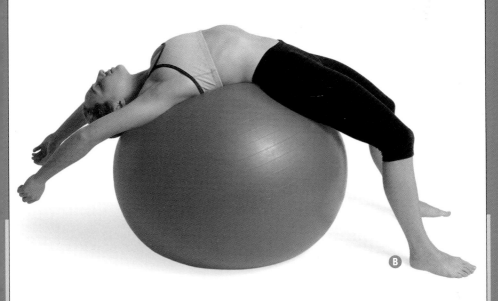

Sölveborn Stretching

In order to correctly apply this particular method, it is necessary to go through three phases:
—Muscle contraction;
—Muscle relaxation;
—Muscle elongation.

In the first phase, the muscle to be stretched must be made to contract (that is, tighten) for 10–30 seconds at maximum intensity, being careful to avoid causing any isometric contractions. In the second phase, the muscle must be made to relax for 2–3 seconds. Thirdly, one must proceed to stretch for 10–30 seconds quite slowly and gradually until maximal extension is reached.

The application of this method requires the same knowledge, theoretical suppositions, and precautions already used for the Anderson method. The Sölveborn method, however, calls for exercise sequences that place more emphasis on skillful execution compared with the exercises presented earlier, which stress the early phases of muscle contraction. The Sölveborn method is therefore appropriate for more experienced athletes, who have a certain store of knowledge, related either to general physiology or to physical training in particular.

We recommend the following sequence of exercises, which are indicated for track. Of course, such a regimen can be applied to other sport disciplines as well, in which the leg muscles and joints play a primary role.

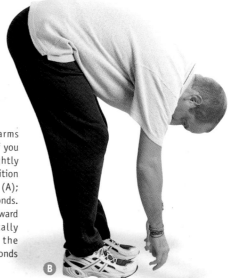

▶ **EXERCISE 1**
Stand with your arms held out in front of you and your legs slightly bent. Hold this position for 10–30 seconds (A); release for 2–3 seconds. Exhale, bending forward and incrementally reaching toward the floor, for 10–30 seconds (B). Repeat.

Ⓐ　　　　Ⓑ

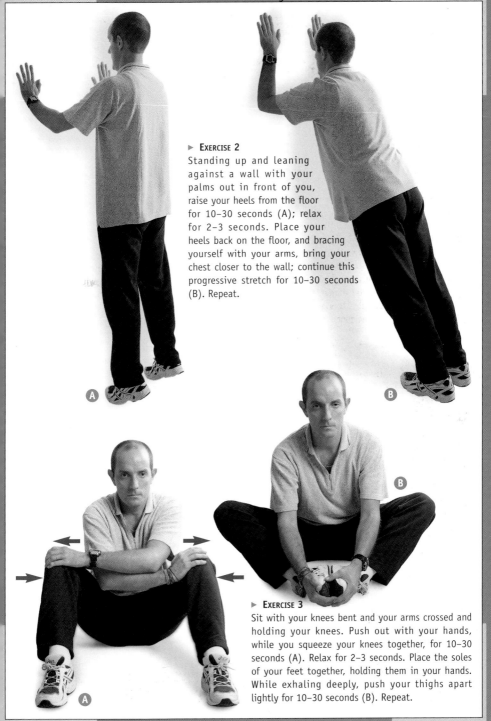

► **EXERCISE 2**
Standing up and leaning against a wall with your palms out in front of you, raise your heels from the floor for 10–30 seconds (A); relax for 2–3 seconds. Place your heels back on the floor, and bracing yourself with your arms, bring your chest closer to the wall; continue this progressive stretch for 10–30 seconds (B). Repeat.

► **EXERCISE 3**
Sit with your knees bent and your arms crossed and holding your knees. Push out with your hands, while you squeeze your knees together, for 10–30 seconds (A). Relax for 2–3 seconds. Place the soles of your feet together, holding them in your hands. While exhaling deeply, push your thighs apart lightly for 10–30 seconds (B). Repeat.

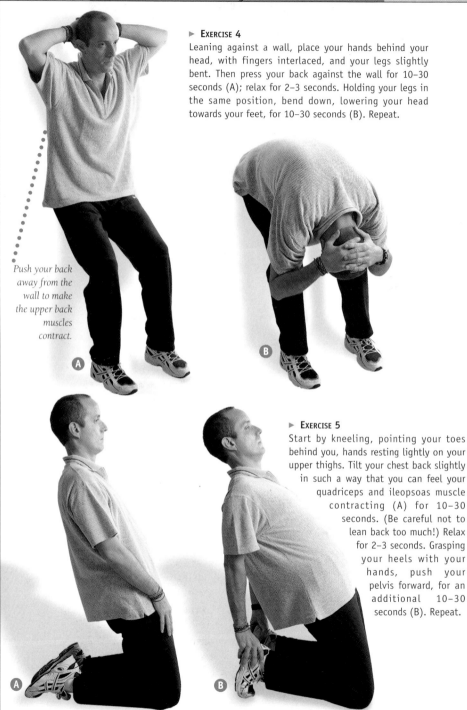

► EXERCISE 4

Leaning against a wall, place your hands behind your head, with fingers interlaced, and your legs slightly bent. Then press your back against the wall for 10–30 seconds (A); relax for 2–3 seconds. Holding your legs in the same position, bend down, lowering your head towards your feet, for 10–30 seconds (B). Repeat.

Push your back away from the wall to make the upper back muscles contract.

A

B

► EXERCISE 5

Start by kneeling, pointing your toes behind you, hands resting lightly on your upper thighs. Tilt your chest back slightly in such a way that you can feel your quadriceps and ileopsoas muscle contracting (A) for 10–30 seconds. (Be careful not to lean back too much!) Relax for 2–3 seconds. Grasping your heels with your hands, push your pelvis forward, for an additional 10–30 seconds (B). Repeat.

A

B

Index